Greek Medical Manuscripts
Diels' Catalogue

Tome 2: Corpus Hippocraticum

Medical Traditions

Edited by
Alain Touwaide

Volume 2/2

De Gruyter

Greek Medical Manuscripts
Diels' Catalogue

Tome 2: Corpus Hippocraticum

Newly revised and updated by
Alain Touwaide

De Gruyter

ISBN 978-3-11-060067-4
e-ISBN (PDF) 978-3-11-060000-1
ISSN 2567-6938

Library of Congress Control Number: 2020945916

Bibliographic information published by the Deutsche Nationalbibliothek
The Deutsche Nationalbibliothek lists this publication in the Deutsche Nationalbibliografie; detailed bibliographic data are available on the Internet at http://dnb.dnb.de.

Cover image: Collage of illustrations in medical treatises from the 1st to the 16th century CE, from Greece and Rome, to the Arabic World and China.

Printing: CPI books GmbH, Leck

www.degruyter.com

Table of contents

Foreword *vii*

Introduction *xi*

Acknowledgements *xxxi*

Indices of Manuscripts

Diels' Location and Shelfmark *xxxiii*

City and Library names

1. Names according to Diels *xxxvii*

2. Standard English names *xxxix*

Manuscripts *xli*

Current Location and Shelfmark *lxi*

City and Library names *lxv*

Manuscripts *lxvii*

Manuscripts of the Corpus Hippocraticum *1*

Foreword

The study of Greek manuscripts of medical content has seen a significant, though not exclusive, investigation by Alain Touwaide, whose life of scholar has been entirely devoted to the knowledge and valorization of the medical traditions of the Mediterranean world with a particular reference to the history of ancient and medieval Greek medicine.

The revisions and updates of the catalogues of Greek medical manuscripts compiled in the early 20th century by an équipe of philologists, guided by the distinguished historian of ancient Greek philosophy and medicine Hermann Diels (*Die Handschriften der antiken Ärzte*), are a cornerstone of Touwaide's scientific research on medical manuscripts, the further developments of which already include plans for a detailed catalogue of all surviving witnesses according to the norms of modern catalography.

Four years after his 2016 voluminous *Census of Greek Medical Manuscripts*, the publication of this new and substantial reference work constitutes a further step, complementary to the previous one, of his programme that will ultimately allow for the critical edition of a series of Greek medical texts in a way reminiscent of the *Corpus Medicorum* conceived by Diels over a century ago as the natural outcome of the catalogues of manuscripts that he coordinated.

If Alain Touwaide embarked on an arduous task with his *Census* and the compilation of an updated list of Greek manuscripts with medical contents—many of which were not listed in Diels' early 20th-century catalogues—the completion of a renewed Diels is a no less demanding endeavour. Diels' catalogues, which have been the reference for over a century for any scholar interested in the study of late antique and medieval Greek medicine from any perspective, are known, indeed, to suffer several limitations—besides the incompleteness of their inventory of manuscripts (well highlighted by the numerous complements provided in the *Census*)—that can be traced to the difficulty in identifying manuscripts generated by Diels' use of shelfmarks which have been made obsolete since by changes in the name of libraries or collections, in ownership, or in the location of collections. To further make research laborious, the printing of Diels' original edition is rather unclear.

Alain Touwaide has chosen to exactly reproduce the substance of Diels' work, even though he significantly intervened with great acumen on the structure, citation format, and presentation of the text, to make its contents more immediately usable and its consultation easier. An innovative organization of data in five tomes (in which the reproduction of Diels' original text in a decidedly more readable form is followed by two different methods of accessing the information, by type of contents—in tomes two through four—and by manuscript—in the fifth and final tome) is accompanied by an articulated system of indices designed to combine the need to reproduce Diels' original text *ad litteram* and the scientific imperative to update and standardize the method of referencing the manuscripts, and also to multiply the keys for searching the texts. In this view, Touwaide's decision to split the list of authors and works is revealing as it allows for the identification of texts by both their Greek and Latin title (albeit following the form, which is not always consistent, of the titles in Diels' original version), thus providing a first effort for a future standardization. Equally inspired by a justifiable need for clarity and simplification is the choice of accompanying the index of the original shelfmarks of manuscripts with a list of the English names of the cities and libraries. Finally, the layout of this renewed Diels clearly improves on the original edition, structuring its presentation in a much clearer and more effective way through different levels of indentation.

Those who are acquainted with Alain Touwaide know that only his visionary and tenacious spirit, supported by an unshakable patience and a truly extraordinary work capacity, could have pushed him to embark alone on the revision of the catalogues that Diels conceived and could complete thanks to the collaboration of a team of no fewer than thirty scholars. Touwaide's revision required many long years of meticulous work, with a sheer quantity of doublechecks, corrections, and identifications of new locations and shelfmarks, as well as *in situ* autoptic inspection of many manuscripts and sometimes even of entire collections.

Though constantly making explicit its connection with Diels' original work through its coherent and functional system of cross-references, the present revision of Diels will ultimately make it unnecessary to refer to the old Diels and make it possible, instead, to work only with updated lists of manuscripts. Furthermore, the multiple indices extremely well designed by Touwaide and the cross-referencing they make possible pave the way to a future, highly desirable transfer of data from a printed form to an open database, much of the necessary material of which is contained in the present work, in addition to the new data already provided by the *Census*. It can be expected that such a database will be constantly expanded and updated by integrating the results of the new developments and research that the catalogue that we have here will undoubtedly contribute to, promote, and generate.

The renewed Diels that we have here deserves to be hailed as an invaluable reference for both the niche of scholars scrutinizing Greek medical manuscripts and texts, and the wider circle of the historians of medicine, pharmacy, and ancient and medieval science, in a way that faithfully reflects the cross-disciplinary approach to the study of medical traditions that Alain Touwaide has convincingly advocated for for years in the name of a fruitful alliance of sciences and the humanities.

We now wish that, as a further contribution to the knowledge of the ancient Greek medical tradition, he will publish a much needed catalogue of Greek medical manuscripts and texts, not only those listed in Diels, but also the many new ones of which he has revealed the existence thanks to his unwavering energy, his devotion to research, and the passion for Greek medicine that has constantly distinguished his life.

Marilena Maniaci
Università degli Studi di Cassino e del Lazio meridionale
Rome, August 2, 2020

Introduction

Just over a century has passed since a team of scholars from across Europe, led by German historian of ancient philosophy and science Hermann Diels (1848–1922)[1], compiled the manuscripts containing Greek medical texts and their medieval translations into a catalogue[2]. Following such classical bibliographies as the *Bibliotheca Graeca* by Johann Albert Fabricius (1668–1736)[3] and the several *Bibliothecae* by Albrecht von Haller (1708–1777)[4], *Diels*, as the catalogue became known, was a landmark in classical and medico-historical scholarship[5]. It was not completely

1 For a broad approach to Diels' multifaceted activity, see for example Calder et al. 1999. All works referred to in this introduction are cited in an abbreviated form (author's last name and year of publication). For the full reference, see the bibliography at pp. xxi–xxx.

2 The catalogue was published in two issues in 1905 and 1906, in the proceedings of Berlin Academy of Science, with a supplement in 1908 in the same series (Diels 1905, 1906a, and 1908, respectively). The 1905 and 1906 issues were published together as a volume in 1906 (Diels 1906b) with a slightly different title (*Die Handschriften der antiken Ärzte, Griechische Abteilung*) which implied that a similar programme would have dealt with the Latin manuscripts. The frontmatter of the second issue (1906a), which provided a general presentation of the programme, the list of the collaborators, and the bibliography, is reproduced as the front matter of this volume with the same pagination as in the first publication. All three issues (1905, 1906a, and 1908) were reprinted in 1970 with an introduction by Fridolf Kudlien (1928–2008) (Kudlien 1970). The translations under consideration were those in Syriac, Arabic, Hebrew, and Latin according to the treatises.
All references to the catalogue here and in the present work comprise two elements: the first identifies the issue of the catalogue (I, II, or N [for *Nachtrag* = Supplement]), and the second (in Arabic numerals) provides the number of the page(s) referred to (e.g., I.22 or N.49). A number in Arabic numerals between parentheses after the second element, such as e.g., II.63 (2), indicates the number of mentions of a manuscript on the same page.

3 Fabricius' *Bibliotheca Graeca* was originally published in 14 volumes between 1705 and 1728, with a second edition started as early as 1708 and pursued until 1754, and also a third edition of Volumes 1 and 2 published in 1718 and 1752, respectively. The whole *Bibliotheca* was further published in a revised edition by Gottlieb Christopher Harles (1738–1815) in 12 volumes published between 1790 and 1809, with an *Index* in 1838. Under the general designation *Bibliotheca Graeca*, all volumes have a distinctive title that indicates their respective contents. In the first volume this title makes an explicit reference to manuscripts (... *notitia Scriptorum Veterum Graecorum quorumcunque monumenta integra, aut fragmenta edita exstant: tum plerorumque è MSS. ac deperditis* ...). On Fabricius, see Verner 1966.

4 The first of Haller's *Bibliothecae* was the *Bibliotheca botanica* (1771–1772), which included large chapters on ancient physicians (see for example, Dioscorides, vol. 1, pp. 79–87 [page 79 is numbered 97]). It was followed by the *Bibliotheca chirurgica* (1774–1775), the *Bibliotheca anatomica* (1774–1777), and the *Bibliotheca medicinae practicae* (1776–1788).

5 For the history of the search for the manuscripts of Greek medical texts from the Renaissance to Diels, see Touwaide 2009, particularly pp. 456–508.

unprecedented, however. From the late eighteenth century on, several similar compilations were made, indeed, but they relied either on earlier literature or on *in situ* inspection of just some collections by single scholars. These were the bibliographies compiled by Johann Christian Gottlieb Ackermann (1756–1801)[6] and the pioneering search for manuscripts by the German scholar Friedrich Reinhold Dietz (1804–1836) in the 1830s[7], followed shortly after by the exploratory missions of the French historian of medicine Charles Daremberg (1817–1872), mostly in England[8], with a similar collection of material *in loco* at the Bibliothèque nationale in Paris by the Greek ophthalmologist Georges Costomiris (1849–1902)[9]. Diels' enterprise was different in its systematicity and scale, in addition to its organization, its team[10], and its international network[11] which combined in-house bibliographical research[12] and *in-*

6 Ackermann's bibliographies with their lists of manuscripts for Hippocrates, Dioscorides and Galen, were published in Harles' edition of Fabricius' *Bibliotheca Graeca* (vol. 2 [1791], pp. 506–611, 4 [1795], pp. 673–702, and 5 [1796], pp. 377–500, respectively). The lists of Hippocratic and Galenic manuscripts were reproduced in the edition of these authors in Kühn's *Medicorum Graecorum Opera quae exstant* under the title *Historia literaria* (for Hippocrates, see vol. 1 [1825], pp. I–CCVI; for Galen, see vol. 1 [1821]), pp. XIX–CCLXV). Interestingly enough, Diels referred to these two lists. The list of manuscripts for Dioscorides, *De materia medica*, in Kühn's *Medicorum Graecorum Opera quae exstant* (see vol. 1 [1829], pp. XX–XXVI) did not reproduce Ackermann's, but was compiled by the editor of the text, Kurt Sprengel (1766–1833).

7 Dietz traveled through Germany, Italy, Spain, France, and Britain, systematically searching for codices containing Greek medical texts (see Dietz 1832: IX–X; Dietz 1834: 1.IV), principally Hippocrates, but also Oribasius (he was supposed to prepare an edition for the corpus edited by Kühn), Aetius, the commentators on Hippocrates, Ioannes Zacharias Actuarius, Greek chemical works, Soranus, Paul of Aegina, Rufus of Ephesus, Erotianus, Nicander, Theophilus, Symeon Seth, and others (e.g., Severus iatrosophist whose treatise he published [Dietz 1836]).

8 See the reports of his travels in Daremberg 1845, 1848, 1851, and 1852, with a reproduction of the last two in the form of a monograph in 1853.

9 Costomiris published the results of his investigations at the Bibliothèque nationale in a series of five contributions to the *Revue des études grecques* published between 1889 and 1897.

10 The collaborators of the program are listed in the front matter of the 1906 issue and the 1906 reprint (p. X) with some further names in the 1908 supplement (p. 23). Besides the collaborators *in loco* (among whom were Ph.D. candidates) coordinated in collaboration by Diels and Johan Ludwig Heiberg (1854–1928), the team included several German scholars as Joseph Heeg (1881–1916) in Munich, Georg Helmreich (1849–1921) in Ansbach, Johannes Ilberg (1860–1930) in Leipzig, Karl Kalbfleich (1868–1946) in Marburg, Iwan von Müller (1830–1917) at that time in Munich, Paul Schwarz (1867–1938), then in Berlin, and Max Wellmann (1863–1933). Their number was higher, however, as the reading of the catalogues indicates: the annotations that accompany the mention of some manuscripts refer to scholars whose name does not appear in the two lists of collaborators.

11 The list of collaborators includes several individuals from abroad who were librarians or academics with a special interest in the history of ancient medicine and medical literature, including translations. These scholars were the following (in alphabetical order of last name): Hartwig (Henry) Derembourg (1844–1908) in Paris; Eduard Gottlob (1856–1922) in Krems a.

situ examination of entire library collections by local scholars or members of Diels' team in mission abroad[13].

Remarkably enough, the vast collection of data contained in the two issues of Diels' catalogues was assembled in barely four years[14], witnessing an exceptional mobilization of efforts and resources[15]. Although a supplement—presented as the first—was published in 1908, it was not followed by any other. Shortly after, the team lost some of its collaborators in the First World War[16], and the systematic search for the manuscripts of ancient medical texts was no longer pursued. Nevertheless, several

---

d. Donau; Montague Rhodes James (1862–1936) in Cambridge; Philip Christian Molhuysen (1870–1944) in Leiden; Alessandro Olivieri (1872–1950) in Naples; Adriano Piccolomini (1843–1907) in Cesena; Anton Ritter von Premerstein (1869–1935) in Vienna; Hans Raeder (1859–1969) in Copenhagen; Walter Scott (1855–1925) in Oxford, with a parenthesis in Montreal (1905–1908); Hermann Schöne (1870–1941) in Basel; Rezső Vári (1867–1940) in Budapest, and Eric Otto Windstedt (1880–1955) in Oxford. This list is not exhaustive, however, as other names appear scattered in the catalogues. The different collaborators interacted as the references to collations (see below) indicate.

12 The consulted bibliography (listed in the 1906a issue [pp. XI–XXIII] with a supplement in 1908 [pp. 23–24]) does not account for the full extent of the library resources consulted by the collaborators of the catalogues, which contain scattered references to works not included in the bibliographical lists.

13 One such mission was that of Max Wellmann, who spent 1906–1907 in Italy, where he particularly investigated the collections of the Vatican and the Marciana libraries. As a result, the 1908 supplement contains multiple annotations made on the basis of his personal consultation of manuscripts.

14 To give an idea of the sheer quantity of data presented in the catalogues, suffice it to say that the number of items from Greek manuscripts only amounts to over 14,000. To this we should add the multiple collations of manuscripts made by the collaborators of the programme during *in loco* research stays or on their behalf that are mentioned in the catalogue. Ilberg, for example, collated himself or received collations of most of the Hippocratic writings from manuscripts at the Vatican Library, and in Florence, Venice, Vienna, and Paris, whereas Helmreich concentrated on Galen (in one case at least, he had a collation of all but one manuscript of a Galenic treatise; see I.83–84).

15 For the history of the programme, see Kollesch 1973, 1989, and 1999; and more recently, Nutton 2004.

16 This was the case of Bruno Rappaport (1875–1915), who managed the data of the catalogues in collaboration with Joahnnes Mewald (1880–1964). On this, see Diels' introductory remarks (*Vorbemerkungen*) to the catalogue (Diels 1906a: pp. I–IX), which include the reports by Rappaport (pp. III–VI) and Mewaldt (pp. VI–VIII). On Rappaport, see the obituary by Regling, 1920. Another victim of the First World War was Joseph Heeg. During the compilation of the catalogues, the program lost another of its members, the orientalist Ludwig Nix (1865–1904) who had collected much material about the Arabic translations of Greek medical works.

editions of Greek medical texts were published thanks to the material collected during the compiling of the catalogues[17].

Addenda and *corrigenda* to Diels[18], studies of the manuscripts or tradition of specific medical treatises[19], and the systematic inventory of the manuscripts of texts to be edited, with the analysis of their tradition[20], punctuated the twentieth-century scholarship devoted to the ancient medical literature. After World War II, an

17 The first such edition was that of Philumenus, *De venenatis animalibus*, by Max Wellmann who discovered the text in the manuscript *Vaticanus graecus* 284 during his research stay at the Vatican Library (Wellmann 1908). This edition, which inaugurated the *Corpus Medicorum Graecorum*, brilliantly illustrated the function of the catalogues as a source of firsthand material for the preparation of the critical editions to be published in the *Corpus*. It is probably significant that it was followed in 1914 by the edition of the Arabic translation of a Pseudo-Galenic treatise by Gotthelf Bergsträsser (1886–1933) (Bergsträsser 1914), and the first edition of Galen in the *Corpus* by three collaborators of the programme (Mewaldt et al. 1914). Another Galenic edition, prepared by another group of three collaborators, followed the next year (Diels et al. 1915), together with Celsus by Friedrich Marx (1869–1941) and, the following year, Quintus Serenus Sammonicus by Friedrich Vollmer (1867–1923). After a short interruption due to World War I, no fewer than 15 editions were published between 1921 and 1937, with one edition every year from 1926 on, including (in chronological order of publication) the vast medical encyclopedias of Paul of Aegina (Heiberg 1921–1924), Oribasius (Raeder 1926, and 1928–1933), and Aetius (*partim*; Olivieri, 1935), in addition to the first Hippocratic edition (Heiberg et al., 1927), Soranus (Ilberg, 1927), Galenic commentaries on Hippocratic treatises (Wenkebach 1934 and 1936) and Galenic works (Koch et al. 1923; De Boer 1937). All this attested to the vitality of the *Corpus* and the usefulness of the catalogue.

18 As early as 1916, Giovanni Mercati (1866–1957), then a *scrittore* at the Vatican Library, published some *addenda* (Mercati 1916, 1917a, and 1917b). Corrections like these are scattered throughout twentieth-century scholarly publications related to the Greek medical literature. Most of them can be found in Touwaide 2016, *passim*, together with new ones. Additions and corrections to Diels' lists of manuscripts of the Latin translations of Greek medical texts have been systematically made, though later. Richard Durling (1932–1999) revised Diels' lists of the Galenic Latin manuscripts (Durling 1967 and 1981, completed only recently by Fortuna and Raia 2006; a cumulative catalogue of the Galenic and Pseudo-Galenic Latin texts [including manuscripts] compiled by Stefania Fortuna and her group is now available online in the form of a constant work in progress [*Galeno. Catalogo delle traduzioni latine*]). Pearl Kibre (1902–1985) compiled new lists of the Hippocratic Latin manuscripts in several installments (1975–1982) followed by a publication in the form of a monographic catalogue in 1985. It may be relevant to note here that Durling expanded his search for Latin medical manuscripts by browsing a collection of material similar to Diels, Kristeller's *Iter Italicum* (Durling 1985–1993).

19 An early work of this type is Ilberg 1911 on Soranus, followed shortly after by Diels 1912 on Galen's commentary on Hippocrates *Prorrheticum*, and Helmreich 1913 on Symeon Seth.

20 The best examples are the introductions to the editions published in the *Corpus Medicorum Graecorum* (which became more developed over time). Their template includes a list of manuscripts, their description, and a detailed philological analysis. Although these introductions focus on identifying the manuscript(s) to be used as a source or sources of the editions, they provide relevant data on codicology and book history.

unprecedented increase in the interest in paleography and codicology[21] soon led to a renewed search for, and study of, manuscripts[22], new catalogues[23], and, more recently, computerized databases allowing for the storage and multi-criteria querying of increasingly larger amounts of information[24], in addition to the digitization of the collections of manuscripts of several libraries across the world[25]. In the field of Greek medical manuscripts and texts, this resulted in the rediscovery or, in some cases, in the true discovery of manuscripts[26], new catalogues of medical manuscripts[27], the history

---

21 In the field of Greek codicology and palaeography, and also textual history, this interest was pioneered by such scholars as Joseph Mogenet (1913–1980), Herbert Hunger (1914–2000), Jean Irigoin (1920–2006), and Paul Canart (1927–2017). It subsequently led to an increased institutionalization of these disciplines illustrated, among others, by a series of international conferences started in 1974 (see *Paléographie,* 1977). For a recent esquisse of the history of codicology and paleography during the twentieth century, see, for example, Touwaide 2010.

22 Whereas the type of research by Alphonse Dain (1896–1964), Paul Henry (1906–1984), Alexander Turyn (1900–1981), and Jean Irigoin on technical texts (Dain 1930, 1933, 1946), Plotin (Henry 1938, 1941), the Greek tragics (Turyn 1943, 1952, 1957) and Pindar (Turyn 1932, and Irigoin 1952), respectively, was relatively rare until then in the academic production, it became more common later. For examples of such a line of investigation, see Eleuteri 1981 on a literary text (Musaeus) and Sonderkamp 1987 on a Greek medical treatise (Theophanes Nonnos/Chrysobalantes).

23 The increase in the publication of catalogues of manuscripts can be best measured by comparing the successive editions of the so-called *Richard* (Richard 1948, 1958, and 1964, followed by such a punctual review of new catalogues as Irigoin 1970, and the major updated editions of *Richard* by Olivier 1995 and 2018).

24 One such database is PINAKES currently hosted and maintained by the Section Grecque of the Institut de Recherche et d'Histoire des Textes (IRHT) of the Centre National de la Recherche Scientifique (CNRS), in Paris. It is built on the basis of the earlier research conducted at the Pontifical Institute of Medieval Studies at University of Toronto by Robert E. Sinkewicz, who compiled available printed catalogues of manuscripts and published the resulting data in the form of microfiches (Sinkewicz and Hayes 1989; Sinkewicz 1990 and 1992). In the matter of medical manuscripts and texts, see the database built on Diels accessible online through the website of the Institute for the Preservation of Medical Traditions. A precursor of this type of database was the catalogue of incipits of Latin medical treatises compiled as early as 1937 by Lynn Thorndike (1882–1965) and Pearl Kibre (1937). After a revised edition published in 1963, this catalogue has been complemented by Linda E. Voigts and Patricia D. Kurtz (Voigts and Kurz 2004), and transformed in digital form (first as a CD-Rom and now as a database consultable online on the site of the University of Missouri Kansas City).

25 See, for example, the site *Gallica*, of the Bibliothèque nationale de France, *teca* of the Biblioteca Medicea Laurenziana in Firenze, *DVL-DigiVatLib* of the Vatican Library, *DigitalBodleian*, *Digitised Manuscripts* of the British Library or, to mention just some, *e-codices* for the manuscripts in Swiss collections. Significantly enough, the most recent release of the site of the *Corpus Medicorum Graecorum* includes links to the digital version of the manuscripts of the authors for which critical editions have been published in the *Corpus*.

26 The most spectacular case has been the discovery of the forgotten manuscript Thessaloniki, Vlatadon 14, which contains a Galenic text which had remained unknown thus far. See Pietrobelli, 2010, for example. For other cases, see, for example, Roselli 2009 ([Hippocrates]) or

of collections of such codices[28], an accrued attention to medical illustration[29], studies of the textual tradition of Greek medical texts[30] or genres[31], the medical production of some regions[32], and new critical editions, particularly from the mid-twentieth century onward[33]. This activity, which also generated a forum in the form of a series of conferences launched by Antonio Garzya (1927–2012) in 1990 and regularly held

---

Perilli 2011 (Galen's Hippocratic lexicon), and Chatzopoulou 2014 and Tselikas 2014 about *iatrosofia*.

27 For some catalogues, see Hunger and Kresten as early as 1969 about the series *medici graeci* of the National Library of Austria in Vienna, and, more recently, Bouras-Vallianatos 2015 about the holdings of the Wellcome Library in London, with a short supplement in Bouras-Vallianatos 2020. A different type of catalogue is that of Formentin 1978, about the libraries of a region.

28 See, for example, Formentin 1997 about the medical manuscripts in the collection of the national library in Naples.

29 A pioneering work in this field was MacKinney 1965, which lists the medieval manuscripts known at that time in several languages with medical illustrations, with some descriptive elements. Recently see Bernabò 2010.

30 For the entire tradition of some works, see, for example (in chronological order of publication), Kudlien 1960 (Hippocrates, *De articulis*), Rivier 1962 (Hippocrates, *De morbo sacro*), and Alexanderson 1963 (Hippocrates, *Prognosticon*) and 1967 (Galen, *De crisibus*). Among the studies in subsequent years, one might cite Morani 1981 (Nemesius) or, more recently, Perilli 1999 (Galen's Hippocratic lexicon). Similar work is being done in Latin, for example by Green 1996 and 1997, on *Trotula*. Research was also devoted to some lesser-known physicians such as Mercurius (see the study by Masullo 2006), or to some segments or manuscripts of the tradition of one or more works. This is the case of Wilson 1987, for example, regarding a group of Galenic manuscripts (the codices copied by Ioannikios), and Petit 2006 on a group of manuscripts in relation with a text ([Galen], *Introductio*).

31 For this type of catalogue, see, for example, Ihm 2002 on medical commentaries (with references to the manuscripts), or Karas 1994, and Tselikas 1995 on *iatrosophia* (Byzantine and later).

32 For Southern Italy, for example, see Ieraci Bio 1989.

33 After an interruption provoked by World War II, the *Corpus Medicorum Graecorum* published anew critical editions as early as 1950 with a predilection for Galen, also including, however, Hippocratic treatises, Aretaeus, Rufus of Ephesus, Aetius, and Leo medicus, and, more recently (from 1983 on), Stephanus of Athens and Johannes of Alexandria. In the 1960s, the French *Collection des universités de France* launched a new Hippocrates (see Joly 1978 for the first volume; the programme has been pursued by Jacques Jouanna) and, very recently, a new Galen (see Boudon 2000 for the first volume). All this in addition to editions in series specifically devoted to the history of ancient and medieval/Byzantine medicine as *Studies in Ancient Medicine* (for example, Dickson 1998 on Stephanus, and Zipser 2009 on Johannes archiater) or, more recently, *Medicine in the Medieval Mediterranean* (Bennett 2016 on hospital formularies) and *Textos Médicos – Ediciones Críticas* (Lamagna 2017 on Johannes Actuarius' Greek translation of Avicenna, *De urinis*). See also such volumes as Pritchet 1975 and 1982 (both on Johannes of Alexandria) or Garzya and Masullo 2004 (on Cassius Iatrosophista). To this, one might add editions of *iatrosofia* (for example, Tselikas and Ilioudis 1995 and 1997, or Clark 2011).

since[34], was accompanied by a transformation in the history of science and the history of the book. While the former moved its focus from the *Great Scientists*[35] to the *histoire vécue*[36], the latter shifted from book production[37] to book use, that is, to reading, studying, annotating, sharing, and collecting[38].

Both transformational trends highlighted limitations of Diels' catalogues: they are devoted to authored works with a focus on the major physicians of classical antiquity and of the period that became defined in the meantime as *Late Antiquity*, that is, the period up to the end of the School of Alexandria in the 7th century A.D[39]. With only some exceptions[40], they omit the multiple small, but no less important, anonymous works, notebooks, and other formularies that give witness to the practice of medicine[41], and also many of the physicians of all epochs (but especially the Byzantine ones, also with some exceptions, however[42]) who have not been credited with such a foundational role as Hippocrates and Galen.

---

34 For the proceedings of the first conference, see Garzya 1992. The conference has been fairly consistently held every four years, alternately in Naples and Paris. The many communications presented in each edition dealt with a great many authors and texts, including lesser known physicians and their treatises. The proceedings were first edited by Antonio Garzya, and then by Garzya in collaboration with Jacques Jouanna before being edited by both, along with Véronique Boudon-Millot and Amneris Roselli.

35 As an example of this historiography, see the monumental encyclopedic *Introduction to the History of Science* (1927–1948) of George Sarton (1884–1956).

36 See, for example, Perrin 1988 on the skin (followed by Herida 1998, on skin in the Hippocratic writings), Rey 1993 on pain, or Dumouchel 1995 on emotions. One might also mention here the development of the history of the body, particularly its specific perception and its representation, including its defects (Fischer 1991).

37 The focus on book production might be best identified by the development of codicology, explicitly formalized as a discipline in its own right during this period (see Dain 1949).

38 On this approach, see, for example, the works of Guglielmo Cavallo, particularly Cavallo 1988 about libraries, and Cavallo and Chartier 1995 on reading, with a panoramic presentation of medieval reading culture. On reading Greek medical literature, more specifically, see, for example, Cavallo 1993 or, more recently, Mondrain 2003.

39 On the chonological span of the catalogues (from the 5th century B.C. to the 7th A.D.), see Bruno Rappaport's report in the 1906 issue, p. III.

40 Some of these exceptions might be the *Excerpta* (or *Excerpta varia*) listed for several authors, as well as the pseudepigraphic literature (mostly Hippocratic and Galenic) (see for example the remedies attributed to, or extracted from the works of, Hippocrates [I.48–49] and Galen [I.132–133]), in addition to some *iatrosophia* of the Ottoman period listed mostly under Hippocrates (I.42), Galen (I.123 and N.38) and Meletius (II.64), but also under Erasistratos (II.36) and Magnus (II.59), besides references to *iatrosophic* literature about Iustus (N.56), Logadius (N.56), Lucas (N.56), and Syncellus (N.66).

41 For such works (hospital formularies), see, for example, Bennett, 2016.

42 These exceptions are the following (in alphabetical order of their names as in Diels) with their reference to Diels: Abraham (II.3; N.42), Antonius Pyropulus (II.15; N.45), Beniaminus (II.22;

A *New Diels* is now a desideratum of the scholarly community[43]. While urgently needed, it would require that Greek medical manuscripts be newly catalogued and their texts accurately identified, building on the twentieth-century classical scholarship briefly presented above and indeed, going even further through a renewed *in situ* autoptic analysis of manuscripts and the reading of their many texts[44]. Whereas codicological analysis would allow for a better approximation of the time or period and place of production of the manuscripts (and also of their texts in some cases), reading and precise identification of all their texts would lead to a more complete and accurate knowledge of medical literature and practice from antiquity to the Renaissance, particularly thanks to the treatises of the period posterior to the 7th century and, for all periods, the multiple anonymous texts of all types not considered in Diels' catalogues.

The present work aims to lead the study of Greek medical manuscripts and literature of the classical and post-classical periods in that direction. While it fundamentally reproduces Diels' lists of Greek manuscripts, it reformats them in different, yet complementary, ways and provides new search tools that may be used for at least two purposes: compiling a catalogue of Greek medical manuscripts that will eventually generate the material necessary for a *New Diels*, and investigating the tradition, reception, and intellectual, and scientific history of Greek medical literature and medicine.

N.46), Cassius iatrosophista (II.22; N.46), Chariton (II.23), Constantinus Meliteniota (II.24; N.47), Damascenus (II.25), Eleutherus (II.35), Esdras propheta (II.37–38; N.50–51), Euphemius Siculus (II.38; N.51), Iacobus Psychrestus (II.50), Ioannes Chumnos (II.52), Ioannes Esdra (II.53), Ioannes episcopus Prisdyanesis (II.54; N.55), Ioannes Staphidaces (II.55; N.55), Leo (II.57; N.56), Manuel Comnenus (N.57), Maximus (Planudes?) (II.62; N.57), Neophytus Prodromenus (II.68; N.60), Nicolaus Myrepsus (II.69; N.60), Nicomedes iatrosophista (II.69), Paulus Nicaeensis (II.81; N.63), Perzoe (II.81), Philippus Xerus (N.63), Photius monachus (II.85),Taronitus (II.100; N.67), Theophilus (II.101–106; N.68), Theophylactus Simocata (II.106; N.68), and Ioannes Zacharias Actuarius (II.108–111; N.69).

43 Some *instrumenta studiorum* that might be considered as partial *New Diels* are already available. One of them is the catalogue of the manuscripts of the Latin translations of Hippocrates compiled by Pearl Kibre (above). Other two are the analytical lists of the manuscripts of the Arabic translations of Greek medical literature and original Arabic medical literature compiled by Sezgin 1970 (medicine, pharmacy, and zoology) and 1971 (alchemy, chemistry, botany, and agriculture), and Ullmann 1970 (medicine). One might also add the inventory of illustrated medical manuscripts compiled by MacKinney as early as 1965 (not only Greek and Latin, but also Syriac, Arabic and Turkish, and the roman languages, English, and German). Relevant also, the bibliographical lists compiled by Gerhard Fichtner (1932–2012) for Hippocrates and Galen (first published on demand, with several successive versions from 1985 on, and now available on line on the website of *Corpus Medicorum Graecorum*).

44 For a proposal in that sense, see Touwaide 2018. Whereas a publication upon completion of the research would be highly desirable, a gradual publication of available data in the form of a work in progress on the Internet might be useful, be it for a catalogue of manuscripts or a *New Diels*.

As such, the present work offers a set of new *instrumenta studiorum* for further developments in manuscript studies, the classical, medical and scientific traditions, and medical history.

Each of the five tomes of the present work has a specific content and purpose. The first tome exactly reproduces Diels' lists of Greek medical manuscripts[45], excluding the lists of the manuscripts containing the possible medieval translations of Greek medical texts into Syriac, Arabic, Hebrew, or Latin according to the treatises. It is not a photographic reproduction of Diels' original pages, however. Whereas lists of manuscripts in the original printing of Diels are presented in the form of blocks of continuous texts, they are rearranged here in the form of enumerations that clearly distinguish each item. The bibliography of Diels has been treated in a similar way for the purposes of clarity. The lists of manuscripts and the bibliography comprise most of the first tome, which is complemented by two indices: one of the authors and texts included in Diels, and the other of the manuscripts listed in Diels. For the purposes of easy and direct consultation, both of these indices open the first tome, which aims to not only make Diels available in a handy format, but to facilitate its use in research.

The remaining four tomes differ with regard to substance and purpose. All of them reproduce the contents of the manuscripts as described in Diels, including all annotations about title, *incipit*, *desinit* and lacunae, in addition to possible similarities with other manuscripts, sources, or copies. They proceed by manuscript (instead of by authors and works as in Diels' original publication). Identification of manuscripts exactly reproduces Diels' elements (city, library, and collection as appropriate, followed by shelfmark). The identification of many manuscripts required updating. This is the case for the several items known in Diels through earlier literature without exact identification. It is also the case of the codices destroyed during the two World Wars of the twentieth century, and of those that have changed location after the publication of Diels. Finally, it is also the case for those manuscripts which have received new shelfmarks. For all of these manuscripts, tomes two through five provide supplementary information with their exact identification, their state of preservation and location, or

45 Until a new reprint is published, Diels does not seem to be widely available (in spite of the 1970 reprint). WorldCat lists only 20 copies across the world. Nevertheless, digital copies are available on the Internet with different levels of quality, accuracy, and completeness via such sites as the *Corpus Medicorum Graecorum*, the Royal College of Physicians (RCP) in London, the Medic@ collection of the BIUSanté in Paris, the Digitale Bibliothek of the Münchener DigitalisierungsZentrum of the Bayerische Staatsbibliothek in Munich, and Google. These copies are linked on some other websites such as the Internet Archive, the UK Medical Heritage Library, the Medical Heritage Library, and European Libraries. As mentioned above, a database built on the basis of Diels is available on the website of the Institute for the Preservation of Medical Traditions.

their new shelfmark[46]. Another contribution of these tomes is their index of manuscripts, which includes possible new locations and shelfmarks, thus allowing one to search for manuscripts in two different, yet complementary ways: by their location and shelfmark as in Diels' time or in present time.

Besides these shared features, tomes two through five differ further by their content. Tomes two through four are each devoted to one author or a group of authors: tome two is devoted to Hippocrates, tome three to Galen, and tome four to the authors defined in Diels as *the remaining physicians* (*Die übrigen griechischen Ärzte ausser Galenos und Hippocrates*), that is, all the other authors of classical and late antiquity, with some Byzantine ones as well[47]. These three volumes aim to allow for a general study of the whole manuscript tradition of the textual bodies they are devoted to. Although they still have a limited documentary basis, they compensate for the lack of relevant instruments in currently available literature, and they provide the substance for first reconstructions of the whole tradition of the treatises by (or attributed to) Hippocrates, Galen, and the other Greek physicians considered by Diels.

Tome five goes further in laying down the basis of what will become a general catalogue of Greek medical manuscripts, as it lists the entire contents of all the manuscripts mentioned in Diels. It proceeds as do tomes two through four, by city and library in alphabetical order and, for each library, by collection and shelfmark, with their new locations and identifications as relevant. It also contains all the descriptive annotations about the texts included in Diels. Like tomes two through four, it contains an index of manuscripts that also lists possible new locations and identifications, allowing one to search for manuscripts on the basis of Diels or by their present location and identification.

By reproducing Diels' inventory of, and data on, Greek medical manuscripts, by rearranging them for new investigations, and by providing them with updated identification and new *instrumenta studiorum*, this work aims to not only make Diels newly available in a handy format with updated information and to expand the range of its applications, but to make further strides in the direction of a general catalogue of Greek medical manuscripts. This catalogue, in turn, will lead to the much needed *New Diels* that may be expected to transform the study and understanding of the Greek medical literature and medicine, with their tradition.

46 For these data, see Touwaide, 2016.

47 For these physicians, see note 42.

Bibliography

Ackermann 1791: Johannes Chr. Ackermann, "Caput XXIII De Hippocrate, Medicorum Principe, et Polybo eius Discipulo", in Ioannes Albertus Fabricius, *Bibliotheca Graeca sive Notitia Scriptorum Veterum Graecorum quorumcumque Monumenta Integra aut Fragmenta edita exstant tum plerorumque e MSS. ac deperditis ab auctore recognita*. Editio quarta variorum curis emendatior atque auctior curante Gottlieb Christophoro Harles. Accedunt B. I. A. Fabricii et Christoph. Augusti Heumanni Supplementa inedita, Volumen secundum. Hamburgi: apud Carolum Ernestum Bohn; Lipsiae: Ex Officina Breitkopfia, 1791, pp. 506–611.

Ackermann 1795: Johannes Chr. Ackermann, "Caput III De Dioscoride", in Ioannes Albertus Fabricius, *Bibliotheca Graeca sive Notitia Scriptorum Veterum Graecorum quorumcumque Monumenta Integra aut Fragmenta edita exstant tum plerorumque e MSS. ac deperditis ab auctore recognita*. Editio tertia variorum curis emendatior atque auctior curante Gottlieb Christophoro Harles. Accedunt Christophori Augusti Heumanni Supplementa inedita, Volumen quartum. Hamburgi: apud Carolum Ernestum Bohn; Lipsiae: Ex Officina Breitkopfia et Haertelia, 1795, pp. 673–702.

Ackermann 1796: Johannes Chr. Ackermann, " Caput XIX (olim XVII) Claudius Galenus", in Ioannes Albertus Fabricius, *Bibliotheca Graeca sive Notitia Scriptorum Veterum Graecorum quorumcumque Monumenta Integra aut Fragmenta edita exstant tum plerorumque e MSS. ac deperditis ab auctore recognita*. Editio tertia variorum curis emendatior atque auctior curante Gottlieb Christophoro Harles. Accedunt Christophori Augusti Heumanni Supplementa inedita, Volumen quintum. Hamburgi: apud Carolum Ernestum Bohn; Lipsiae: Ex Officina Breitkopfia et Haertelia, 1796, pp. 377–500.

Ackermann 1821: Johannes Chr. Ackermann, "Historia literaria Claudii Galeni ... ex Jo. Alb. Fabricii Biblioth. Graec. ex ed. Gli. Cph. Harles, vol. V. P. 377–500", in Carolus Gottlob Kühn (ed.), *Claudii Galeni Opera omnia*, Tomus 1 (Medicorum Graecorum Opera quae exstant 1). Leipzig: Carl Cnobloch, 1821, pp. XVII–CCLXV.

Ackermann 1825: Johannes Chr. Ackermann, "Historia literaria Hippocratis ... ex Jo. Alb. Fabricii Biblioth. Graec. ex edit. Gli. Cph. Harles, vol. II. P. 506–511. Desunta et hinc inde aucta et emendata", in Carolus Gottlob Kühn (ed.), *Magni Hippocratis Opera omnia*, Tomus 1 (Medicorum Graecorum Opera quae exstant 21). Leipzig: Carl Cnobloch, 1825, pp. I–CCVI).

Alexanderson 1963: Bengt Alexanderson, *Die Hippokratische Schrift Prognostikon. Überlieferung and Text* (Studia Graeca et Latina Gothoburgensia 17). Göteborg: Acta Universitatis Gothoburgensis, 1963.

Alexanderson 1967: Bengt Alexanderson, *Galenos, Περὶ κρίσεων. Uberlieferung und Text* (Studia Graeca et Latina Gothoburgensia 23). Göteborg: Acta Universitatis Gothoburgensis, 1967.

Bennett 2016: David Bennett, *Medicine and Pharmacy in Byzantine Hospitals. A study of the extant formularies* (Medicine in the Medieval Mediterranean 7). London and New York, NY: Routledge, 2016.

Bersgträsser 1914: Gotthelf Bergsträsser (ed.), *Pseudogaleni in Hippocratis de septimanis* (Corpus Medicorum Graecorum XI 2,1). Lipsiae et Berolini: B.G. Teubner, 1914.

Bernabò 2010: Massimo Bernabò (ed.), *La collezione di testi chirurgici di Niceta. Firenze, Biblioteca Medicea Laurenziana, plut. 74.7. Tradizione medica classica a Bisanzio* (Folia Picta. Manoscritti miniati medievali 2). Roma: Storia e Letteratura, 2010.

Boudon 2000: Véronique Boudon, *Galien*, Tome II: *Exhortation à l'étude de la médecine. Art médical.* Texte établi et traduit (Collection des Universités de France). Paris: Belles Lettres, 2000.

Bouras-Vallianatos 2015: Petros Bouras-Vallianatos, "Greek Manuscripts at the Wellcome Library in London: A Descriptive Catalogue", *Medical History* 59 (2015), pp. 275–326.

Bouras-Vallianatos 2020: Petros Bouras-Vallianatos, "Addenda et Corrigenda to the 'Greek Manuscripts at the Wellcome Library in London: A Descriptive Catalogue', *Medical History* 59 (2015): 275–326", in Petros Bouras-Vallianatos (ed.), *Exploring Greek Manuscripts in the Library at Wellcome Collection in London*. London: Routledge, 2020, pp. 181–182.

Calder et al. 1999: William M. Calder III, and Jaap Mansfeld (eds.), with the participation of Alex Leukart, François Paschould, and Olivier Reverdin, *Hermann Diels (1848–1922) et la science de l'Antiquité. Huit exposés suivis de discussion ... Vandoeuvres-Genève, 17–21 août 1998* (Entretiens sur l'Antiquité classique 45). Genève: Fondation Hardt, 1999.

Cavallo 1988: Guglielmo Cavallo, *Le biblioteche nel mondo antico e medievale* (Biblioteca universale Laterza 250). Bari and Roma: Laterza, 1988.

Cavallo 1993: Guglielmo Cavallo, "Libri di medicina: gli usi di un sapere", in Evelyne Patlagean (ed.), *Maladie et société à Byzance* (Collectanea 3). Spoleto: Centro italiano di studi sull'alto medioevo, 1993, pp. 43–56.

Cavallo and Chartier 1995: Guglielmo Cavallo and Roger Chartier (eds), *Storia della lettura nel mondo occidentale* (Storia e Società). Bari and Roma: Laterza, 1995.

Chatzopoulou 2014: Βενετία Χατζοπούλου, "Δύο ἄγνωστα ἰατρικὰ χειρόγραφα μὲ ἔργα τοῦ Νικολάου Βελισδονίτη", in Παναγιώτης Βλάχος, *Όσιος Ευγένιος ο Αιτωλός και αι Σχολαί των Αγράφων κατά την Τουρκοκρατία. Καρπενήσιον, 7–9 Όκτωβρίου 2011. Πρακτικά.* Αθήνα: Σύνδεσμος "Ευγένιος ο Αιτωλός", 2014, vol. 2, pp. 573–581.

Clark 2011: Patricia A. Clark, *A Cretan Healer's Handbook in the Byzantine Tradition: Text, Translation and Commentary* (Medicine in the Medieval Mediterranean 3). Aldershot, and Burlington, VT: Ashgate, 2011.

Costomiris 1889: Georges A. Costomiris, "Etudes sur les écrits inédits des anciens médecins grecs et ceux dont le texte original est perdu, mais qui existent en latin ou en arabe. Première série: Hippocrate, Cratevas, Aelius Promotus, Galien", *Revue des études grecques* 1 (1889), pp. 343–383.

Costomiris 1890: Georges A. Costomiris, "Etudes sur les écrits inédits des anciens médecins grecs et ceux dont le texte original est perdu, mais qui existent en latin ou en arabe. Deuxième série: L'Anonyme de Daremberg, Métrodora, Aétius", *Revue des études grecques* 3 (1890), pp. 145–179.

Costomiris 1891: Georges A. Costomiris, "Etudes sur les écrits inédits des anciens médecins grecs et ceux dont le texte original est perdu, mais qui existent en latin ou en arabe. Troisième série: Alexandre (Sophiste et Roi), Timothée, Léon le Sophiste, Théophane Nonnos, les Ephodes", *Revue des études grecques* 4 (1891), pp. 97–110.

Costomiris 1892: Georges A. Costomiris, "Études sur les écrits inédits des anciens médecins grecs. Quatrième série: Hippiatriques et auteurs du XIe siècle: Psellus, Siméon Seth, Damnastès", *Revue des études grecques*, 5 (1892), pp. 61–72.

Costomiris 1897: Georges A. Costomiris, "Etudes sur les écrits inédits des anciens médecins grecs et ceux dont le texte original est perdu, mais qui existent en latin ou en arabe. Cinquième série: XIIIe–XIVe siècles, Jean Tzetzès, Nicolas Myrepsus, Jean Actuarius", *Revue des études grecques* 10 (1897), pp. 405–445.

Dain 1930: Alphonse Dain, *Les manuscrits d'Onesandros* (Collection d'études anciennes). Paris: Belles Lettres, 1930.

Dain 1933: Alphonse Dain, *La tradition du texte d'Héron de Byzance* (Collection d'études anciennes). Paris: Belles Lettres, 1933.

Dain 1946: Alphonse Dain, *Histoire du texte d'Élien le Tacticien des origines à la fin du moyen âge* (Collection d'études anciennes). Paris: Belles Lettres, 1946.

Dain 1949: Alphonse Dain, *Les manuscrits*. Paris: Belles Lettes, 1949.

Daremberg 1845: Charles Daremberg, "Rapport adressé à M. le Ministre de l'Instruction Publique par .. chargé d'une mission médico-littéraire en Allemagne" *Journal général de l'Instruction publique* 14, no. 33 (23 avril 1845), pp. 193–196, and no. 34 (26 avril 1845), pp. 198–202 (also printed as a booklet under the same title, in Paris, P. Dupont, 15 avril 1845, 32 p.).

Daremberg 1848: Charles Daremberg, "Résumé d'un voyage médico-littéraire en Angleterre. Lu à l'Académie des inscriptions et belle-lettres, dans la séance du 6 octobre", *Gazette médicale de Paris*, 4 novembre 1848, pp. 3–18.

Daremberg 1851: Charles Daremberg, "Notices et extraites des manuscrits médicaux d'Angleterre", *Archives des Missions scientifiques et littéraires*, 1851,VII, VIII, and IX.

Daremberg 1852: Charles Daremberg, "Notices et extraites des manuscrits médicaux d'Angleterre", *Archives des Missions scientifiques et littéraires* 1852, I.

Daremberg 1853: Charles Daremberg, *Notices et extraits des manuscrits médicaux grecs, latins et français, des principales bibliothèques de l'Europe, I: Manuscrits grecs d'Angleterre suivis d'un fragment de Gilles de Corbeil et de scolies inédites sur Hippocrate*. Paris: Imprimerie impériale, 1853.

De Boer 1937: Wilko De Boer (ed.), *Galeni De propriorum animi cuiuslibet dignotione et curatione. De animi cuiuslibet peccatorum dignotione et curatione. De atra bile* (Corpus Medicorum Graecorum V 4, 1. 1). Lipsiae et Berolini: B. G. Teubner, 1937.

Dickson 1998: Keith Dickson (ed.), *Stephanus the Philosopher and Physician, Commentary on Galen's Therapeutics to Glaucon* (Studies in Ancient Medicine 19). Leiden, Boston, MA, Köln: Brill, 1998.

Diels 1905: Hermann Diels (ed.), *Die Handschriften der antiken Ärzte. I. Teil. Hippokrates und Galenos. Im Auftrage der akademischen Kommission herausgegeben* (Abhandlungen der Königlich Preussischen Akademie der Wissenschaften vom Jahre 1905, Philosophisch-historische Klasse, Abhandlung III). Berlin: Königliche Akademie der Wissenschaften, 1905.

Diels 1906a: Hermann Diels, *Die Handschriften der antiken Ärzte. II. Teil. Die übrigen griechischen Ärzte ausser Hippokrates und Galenos. Im Auftrage der akademischen Kommission herausgegeben von -* (Abhandlungen der Königlich Preussischen Akademie der Wissenschaften vom Jahre 1906, Philosophisch-historische Klasse, Abhandlung I). Berlin: Königliche Akademie der Wissenschaften, 1906.

Diels 1906b: Hermann Diels, *Die Handschriften der antiken Ärzte. Griechische Abteilung. Im Auftrage der akademischen Kommission herausgegeben von - aus den Abhandlungen der Königlich Preussischen Akademie der Wissenschaften der Jahre 1905 und 1906*. Berlin: Königliche Akademie der Wissenschaften, 1906.

Diels 1908: Hermann Diels, *Bericht über den Stand des interakademischen Corpus Medicorum Antiquorum und Erster Nachtrag zu den in den Abhandlungen 1905 und 1906 veröffentlichten Katalogen: Die Handschriften der antiken Ärzte. I. und II. Teil. Zusammengestellt im Namen der Kommission der Königlich Preussischen Akademie der Wissenschaften von -* (Abhandlungen der Königlich Preussischen Akademie der Wissenschaften vom Jahre 1907, Philosophisch-historische Klasse, Abhandlung II). Berlin: Königliche Akademie der Wissenschaften, 1908.

Diels 1912: Hermann Diels, *Die handschriftliche Überlieferung des galenischen Commentars zum Prorrheticum des Hippocrates* (Abhandlungen der Königlich Preussischen Akademie der Wissenschaften vom Jahre 1912, Philosophisch-historische Klasse, Abhandlung I). Berlin: Königliche Akademie der Wissenschaften, 1912.

Diels et al. 1915: Hermann Diels (ed.), *Galeni, In Hippocratis Prorrheticum I commentaria III*; Johannes Mewaldt (ed.), *Galeni, De comate secundum Hippocratem*; Josef Heeg (ed.), *Galeni, In Hippocratis Prognosticum commentaria III* (Corpus Medicorum Graecorum V 9, 2). Lipsiae et Berolini: B. G. Teubneri, 1915.

Dietz 1832: Friedrich Reinhold Dietz, *Galeni de dissectione musculorum et de consuetudine libri. Ad fidem codicum manuscriptorum alterum secundum, primum alterum graece edidit.* Lipsiae: Leopold Voss, 1832.

Dietz 1834: Friedrich Reinhold Dietz, *Apollonii Citiensis, Stephani, Palladii, Theophili, Meletii, Damasci, Ioannis aliorum Scholia in Hippocratem et Galenum e codicibus mss. Vindobonens. Monacens. Florentin. Mediolanens. Escorialens. etc. primum graece edidit*, 2 volumes. Regimontii Prussorum: apud fratres Borntraeger, 1834.

Dietz 1836: Friedrich Reinhold Dietz, *Severi Iatrosophistae De clysteribus liber. Ad Fidem Codicis Manuscripti unici Florentini primum Graece edidit.* Regimontii Prussorum: apud Fratres Borntraeger, 1836.

Dumouchel 1995: Paul Dumouchel, *Emotions. Essai sur le corps et le social* (Collection Les Empêcheurs de penser en rond). Le Plessis-Robinson: Synthélabo, 1995.

Durling 1967: Richard J. Durling, "Corrigenda and addenda to Diels' Galenica. I. Codices Vaticani". *Traditio* 23 (1967), pp. 461–476.

Durling 1981: Richard J. Durling, "Corrigenda and addenda to Diels' Galenica. II. Codices Miscellanei". *Traditio* 37 (1981), pp. 373–381.

Durling 1985–1993: Richard J. Durling, "A Guide to the Medical Manuscripts Mentioned in Kristeller's *Iter Italicum*", *Traditio* 41 (1985), pp. 341–365; 44 (1988), pp. 485–536; 46 (1991), pp. 347–379; 48 (1993), pp. 253–316.

Eleuteri 1981: Paolo Eleuteri, *Storia della tradizione manoscritta di Museo* (Biblioteca di Studi Antichi 30). Pisa: Giardini, 1981.

Fabricius 1705–1728: Jo. Alberti Fabricii, *Bibliotheca Graeca* ... Hamburgi: Sumptu Christiani Lievezeit, Typis Spiringlanis, 1705–1728, 14 volumes (after the general title as above, each volume has a specific subtitle that details its contents).

Fabricius ed. Harles 1790–1838: Gottlieb Christophorus Harles, *Ioannis Alberti Fabricii ... Bibliotheca Graeca sive notitia scriptorum veterum graecorum quorumcunque monumenta integra aut fragmenta edita exstant tum plerorumque e MSS. ac deperditis ab auctore tertium recognita et plurimis locis aucta editio quarta variorum curis emendatior atque auctior ... Accedunt B. I. A. Fabricii et Christoph. Augusti Heumanni supplementa inedita.* Hamburgi: apud Carolum Ernestum Bohn; Lipsiae: ex Officina Breitkoppia, 1790–1838, 13 volumes.

Fichtner 1985a: Gerhard Fichtner, *Corpus Galenicum. Verzeichnis der galenischen und pseudogalenischen Schriften.* Tübingen: the author, 1985.

Fichtner 1985b: Gerhard Fichtner, *Corpus Hippocraticum. Verzeichnis der hippokratischen und pseudohippokratischen Schriften.* Tübingen: the author, 1985.

Fischer 1991: Jean-Louis Fischer, *Monstres. Histoire du corps et de ses défauts.* Paris: Syros Alternatives, 1991.

Formentin 1978: Mariarosa Formentin, *I codici greci di medicina nelle tre Venezie* (Università di Padova, Studi bizantini e neogreci 10). Padova: Liviana editrice, 1978.

Formentin 1997: Maria Rosa Formentin, "Codici greci di medicina nella Biblioteca Nazionale Vittorio Emanuele III di Napoli: le vie di acquisizione", in Sergio Sconocchia and Lucio Toneatto (eds.), in collaboration with Daria Crismani, Michele Faraguna, and Italo Pin, *Lingue tecniche del greco e del latino II. Atti del II Seminario internazionale sulla letteratura scientifica e tecnica greca e latina (Trieste, 4–5 ottobre 1993).* Bologna: Pàtron, 1997, pp. 208–216.

Fortuna and Raia 2006: Stefania Fortuna and Annamaria Raia, "Corrigenda and Addenda to Diels *Galenica* by Richard J. Durling: III. Manuscripts and Editions", *Traditio* 61 (2006), pp. 1–30.

Garzya 1992: Antonio Garzya (ed.), *Tradizione e ecdotica dei testi medici tardo-antichi e bizantini. Atti del Convegno internazionale, Anacapri, 29–31 ottobre 1990* (Collectanea 5). Napoli: D'Auria, 1992.

Garzya and Masullo 2004: Antonio Garzya and Rita Masullo (eds), *I problemi di Cassio Iatrosofista. Testo critico, introduzione, apparato critico, traduzione e note*. Napoli: Accademia Pontaniana, 2004.

Green 1996: Monica H. Green, "A Handlist of the Latin and Vernacular Manuscripts of the So-Called Trotula Texts. Part I: The Latin Manuscripts", *Scriptorium* 50 (1996), pp. 137–175.

Green 1997: Monica H. Green, "A Handlist of the Latin and Vernacular Manuscripts of the So-Called Trotula Texts. Part II: The Vernacular Texts and Latin Re-Writings", *Scriptorium* 51 (1997), pp. 80–104.

Haller 1771–1772: Albrecht von Haller, *Bibliotheca botanica qua scripta ad rem herbariam facientia a rerum initiis recensentur*, 2 volumes. Tiguri: Orell, Gessner, Fuessli, et Socc., 1771–1772.

Haller 1774–1775: Albrecht von Haller, *Bibliotheca chirurgica qua scripta ad artem chirurgicam facientia a rerum initiis recensentur*, 2 volumes. Bernae: Em. Haller; Basileae: Joh. Schweighauser, 1774–1775.

Haller 1774–1777: Albrecht von Haller, *Bibliotheca anatomica qua scripta ad anatomen et physiologiam facientia a rerum initiis recensentur*, 2 volumes. Tiguri: Orell, Gessner, Fuessli, et Socc., 1774–1777.

Haller 1776–1788: Albrecht von Haller, *Bibliotheca medicinae practicae qua scripta ad partem medicinae practicam facientia a rerum initiis ad A. MDCCLXXV recensentur*, 4 volumes. Basileae: Joh. Schweighauser, and Bernae: Em. Haller, 1776–1788.

Heiberg 1921–1924: Johannes L. Heiberg (ed.), *Paulus Aegineta*, 2 volumes (Corpus Medicorum Graecorum IX 1–2). Lipsiae et Berolini: B. G. Teubner, 1921–1924.

Heiberg et al. 1927: Johannes L. Heiberg, Johannes Mewaldt, Ernst Nachmanson, Hermann Schoene (eds), *Hippocratis opera: Indices librorum, Iusiurandum, Lex, De arte, De medico, De decente habitu, Praeceptiones, De prisca medicina, De aere locis aquis, De alimento, De liquidorum usu, De flatibus* (Corpus Medicorum Graecorum I 1). Lipsiae et Berolini: B. G. Teubner, 1927.

Helmreich 1913: Georg Helmreich, *Handschriftliche Studien zu Symeon Seth* (Programm des K. humanistischen Gymnasiums in Ansbach für das Schuljahr 1912/13). Ansbach: C. Brügel & Sohn, 1913.

Henry 1938: Paul Henry, *Études Plotiniennes I. Les Etats du texte de Plotin* (Museum Lessianum, Section Philosophique, no 20). Paris: Desclée de Brouwer et Cie; Bruxelles: L'Edition Universelle, 1938.

Henry 1941: Paul Henry, *Études Plotiniennes II. Les Manuscrits des Ennéades* (Museum Lessianum, Section Philosophique 21). Bruxelles: L'Edition Universelle; Paris: Desclée de Brouwer et Cie, and A. et J. Picard, 1941.

Herida 1998: Magid Herida, *La peau dans les écrits hippocratiques* (Thèse de médecine). Paris: Université Paris 6, 1998.

Hunger and Kresten 1969: Herbert Hunger, and Otto Kresten, *Katalog der griechischen Handschriften der Österreichischen Nationalbibliothek*, Teil 2: *Codices juridici, codices medici* (Museion, Veröffentlichungen der Österreichischen Nationalbibliothek, Neue Folge, Vierte Reihe: Veröffentlichungen der Handschriftensammlung, Erster Band: Katalog der griechischen Handschriften der Österreichischen Nationalbibliothek, Teil 2). Wien: Georg Prachner, 1969.

Ieraci Bio 1989: Anna Maria Ieraci Bio, "La trasmissione della letteratura medica greca nell'Italia meridionale fra X e XV secolo", in Antonio Garzya (ed.), *Contributi alla cultura greca nell'Italia meridionale* (Hellenica et Byzantina Neapolitana 13). Napoli: Bibliopolis, 1989, pp. 133–257.

Ihm 2002: Sibylle Ihm, *Clavis Commentariorum der antiken medizinischen Texte* (Clavis Commentariorum Antiquitatis et Medii Aevi 1). Leiden, Boston and Köln: Brill, 2002.

Ilberg 1911: Johannes Ilberg, *Die Überlieferung der Gynäkologie des Soranos von Ephesos* (Abhandlungen der philologisch-historischen Klasse der Königl. Sächsischen Gesellschaft der Wissenschaften Bd. 28, Abhandlung 2). Leipzig: B. G. Teubner, 1911.

Ilberg 1927: Ioannes Ilberg (ed.), *Soranus* (Corpus Medicorum Graecorum IV). Lipsiae et Berolini: B. G. Teubner, 1927.

Irigoin 1952: Jean Irigoin, *Histoire du Texte de Pindare* (Etudes et Commentaires 13). Paris: Klincksieck, 1952.

Irigoin 1970: Jean Irigoin, "Les manuscrits grecs. I. Quelques catalogues récents", *Revue des études grecques* 83 (1970), pp. 500–529.

Joly 1978: Robert Joly, *Hippocrate. Oeuvres complètes*, Tome XIII: *Les lieux dans l'homme. Du système des glandes. Des fistules. Des hémorrhoïdes. De la vision. Des chairs. De la dentition.* Texte établi et traduit (Collection des Universités de France). Paris: Belles Lettres, 1978.

Karas 1994: Γιάννης Καράς, *Οι επιστήμες στην Τουρκοκρατία. Χειρόγραφα και έντυπα*, Τόμος Γ': Οι επιστήμες της ζώης. Παράρτημα. Έργα γενικόν γνωσέων (Κέντρο Νεοελληνικών Ερευνών, Έθνικό Ίδρυμα Ερευνών 48). Αθήνα: Βιβλιοπωλείον της «Εστίας», 1994.

Kibre 1975–1982: Pearl Kibre, "Hippocrates Latinus. Repertorium of Hippocratic Writings in the Latin Middle Ages", *Traditio* 31 (1975), pp. 99–126; 32 (1976), pp. 257–292; 33 (1977), pp. 253–295; 34 (1978), pp. 193–226; 35 (1979), pp. 273–302; 36 (1980), pp. 347–392; 37 (1981), pp. 267–289; 38 (1982), pp. 165–192.

Kibre 1985: Pearl Kibre, *Hippocrates Latinus. Repertorium of Hippocratic Writings in the Latin Middle Ages.* Revised Edition. New York: Fordham University Press, 1985.

Koch et al. 1923: Konrad Koch (ed.), *Galeni, De sanitate tuenda libri VI*; Georg Helmreich (ed.), *Galeni, De alimentorum facultatibus libri III*; *Galeni, De bonis malisque sucis lber*; Karl Kalbfleisch (ed.), *Galeni, De victu attenuante*; Otto Hartlich (ed.), *Galeni, De ptisana* (Corpus Medicorum Graecorum V 4, 2). Lipsiae et Berolini: B. G. Teubner, 1923.

Kollesch 1973: Jutta Kollesch, "Hermann Diels in seiner Bedeutung für die Geschichte der antiken Medizin", *Philologus* 117 (1973), pp. 278–283.

Kollesch 1989: "Die Erschliessung der antiken medizinischen Texte und ihre Probleme – das *Corpus Medicorum Graecorum et Latinorum*", *Gesnerus* 46 (1989), pp. 195–210.

Kollesch 1999: "Die Organisation und Herausgabe des *Corpus Medicorum Graecorum*: ergänzenden Details aus der Korrespondenz zwischen Hermann Diels und Johannes Mewaldt", in William M. Calder III, and Jaap Mansfeld (eds.), with the participation of Alex Leukart, François Paschould, and Olivier Reverdin, *Hermann Diels (1848–1922) et la science de l'Antiquité. Huit exposés suivis de discussion ... Vandoeuvres-Genève, 17–21 août 1998* (Entretiens sur l'Antiquité classique 45). Genève: Fondation Hardt, 1999, pp. 207–223.

Kudlien 1960: Fridolf Kudlien, *Die handschriftliche Überlieferung des Galenkommentars zu Hippokrates de articulis* (Deutsche Akademie der Wissenschaften zu Berlin, Schriften der Sektion für Altertumswissenschaft 27). Berlin: Akademie Verlag, 1960.

Kudlien 1970: Fridolf Kudlien (ed.), *Hermann Alexander Diels, Die Handschriften der antiken Ärzte. I Hippokrates und Galenos II Die übrigen griechische Ärzte III Nachtrag.* Mit einem Vorwort. Leipzig: Zentralantiquariat der deutschen demokratischen Republik, 1970.

Kühn 1821: Karl Gottlieb Kühn (ed.), *Claudii Galeni Opera omnia*, Tomus I (Medicorum graecorum opera quae exstant 1). Lipsiae: Cnobloch, 1821.

Kühn 1825: Karl Gottlieb Kühn (ed.), *Magni Hippocratis Opera omnia*, Tomus I (Medicorum graecorum opera quae exstant 21). Lipsiae: Cnobloch, 1825.

Lamagna 2017: Mario Lamagna, *Giovanni Attuario, L'eccellente trattato sulle urine di Avicenna.* Introduzione, testo critico, traduzione e note al testo (Serie Textos Médicos – Ediciones Críticas.

Ediciones críticas de la Escuela de traductores de Toledo 21). Cuenca: Ediciones de la Universidad de Castilla-La Mancha, 2017.

MacKinney 1965: Loren MacKinney, *Medical Illustrations in Medieval Manuscripts* (Publications of the Wellcome Historical Medical Library, New Series, V). London: Wellcome Historical Medical Library, 1965.

Marx 1915: Fridericus Marx (ed.), *A. Cornelii Celsi quae supersunt* (Corpus Medicorum Latinorum I). Lipsiae et Berolini: In aedibus B. G. Teubneri, 1915.

Masullo 2006: Rita Masullo, "Sul ΠΕΡΙ ΣΦΥΓΜΩΝ attribuito a Mercurio Monaco", in Véronique Boudon-Millot, Antonio Garzya, Jacques Jouanna, and Amneris Roselli (eds.), *Ecdotica e ricezione dei testi medici greci. Atti del V Convegno Internazionale Napoli, 1–2 ottobre 2004* (Collectanea 24). Napoli: M. D'Auria, 2006, pp. 335–346.

Mewaldt et al. 1914: Johannes Mewaldt (ed.), *Galeni, In Hippocratis De natura hominis commentaria III*; Georg Helmreich (ed.), *Galeni, In Hippocratis De victu acutorum commentaria IV*; Johann Westenberger (ed.), *Galeni, De diaeta Hippocratis in morbis acutis* (Corpus Medicorum Graecorum V 9, 1). Lipsiae et Berolini: B. G. Teubner, 1914.

Mercati 1916: Giovanni Mercati, "Minuzie. – 6–8. Pretesi scritti di Paolo l'Egineta e di Galeno. – 9–11. Pretesi scritti di medicina greca", *Bessarione* 32 (1916), pp. 208–211 (reprinted in Giovanni Mercati, *Opere minori raccolte in occasione del settantesimo natalizio sotto gli auspicii di S. S. Pio XI*, vol. 3 [1907–1916] (Studi e Testi 780. Città del Vaticano: Biblioteca Apostolica Vaticana, 1937, pp. 521–524).

Mercati 1917a: Giovanni Mercati, "Minuzie. – 13–17. Altre correzioni ed aggiunte all'op. Die Handschriften der antiken Aerzte. – 18. Per Aezio", *Bessarione* 38 (1917), pp. 50–55 (reprinted in Giovanni Mercati, *Opere minori raccolte in occasione del settantesimo natalizio sotto gli auspicii di S. S. Pio XI*, vol. 4 [1917–1936] (Studi e Testi 79). Città del Vaticano: Biblioteca Apostolica Vaticana, 1937, pp. 16–21).

Mercati 1917b: Giovanni Mercati, "I. Filippo Xeros Reggino, Giovanni Alessandrino iatrosofista e altri nel codice Vaticano degli Ephodia, and II. Un nuovo capitolo di Sorano e tre nuove ricette superstiziose in Aezio", in Giovanni Mercati, *Notizie varie di antica letteratura medica e di bibliografia* (Studi e Testi 31). Roma: Tipografia Poliglotta Vaticana, 1917, pp. 9–41, and 42–46.

Mondrain 2003: Brigitte Mondrain, "Comment était lu Galien à Byzance dans la première moitié du XVe siècle? Contribution à quelques aspects de l'histoire des textes", in Antonio Garzya and Jacques Jouanna (eds), *Trasmissione e ecdotica dei testi medici greci. Atti del IV Convegno internazionale, Parigi 17–19 maggio 2001* (Collectanea 21). Napoli: D'Auria, 2003, pp. 361–384.

Morani 1981: Moreno Morani, *La tradizione manoscritta del "De natura hominis" di Nemesio* (Scienze filologiche e letteratura 18). Milano: Vita e pensiero, 1981.

Nutton 2004: Vivian Nutton, "Ancient Medicine: From Berlin to Baltimore", in Frank Huisman, and John Harley Warner (eds), *Locating Medical History. The Stories and Their Meanings*. Baltimore, MD, and London: Johns Hopkins University Press, 2004, pp. 115–138.

Olivier 1995: Jean-Marie Olivier, *Répertoire des bibliothèques et des catalogues de manuscrits grecs de Marcel Richard. Troisième édition entièrement refondue* (Corpus Christianorum). Turnhout: Brepols, 1995.

Olivier 2018: Jean-Marie Olivier, *Supplément au répertoire des bibliothèques et des catalogues de manuscrits grecs*, 2 volumes (Corpus Christianorum). Turnhout: Brepols, 2018.

Olivieri 1935: Alessandro Olivieri (ed.), *Aetii Amideni Libri medicinales I–IV* (Corpus Medicorum Graecorum VIII 1). Lipsiae et Berolini: B. G. Teubner, 1935.

***Paléographie* 1977:** *La paléographie grecque et byzantine: actes du colloque international sur la paléographie grecque et byzantine organisé dans le cadre des colloques internationaux du Centre*

National de la recherche scientifique, Paris du 21 au 25 octobre 1974 (Issue 559 of Colloques internationaux du Centre National de la Recherche Scientifique 559). Paris: Editions du CNRS, 1977.

Perilli 1999: Lorenzo Perilli, "La tradizione manoscritta del Glossario ippocratico di Galeno (e l'ordinamento alfabetico delle glosse)", in Antonio Garzya, and Jacques Jouanna (eds.), *I testi medici greci. Tradizione e ecdotica. Atti del III Convegno Internazionale, Napoli 15–18 ottobre 1997.* Napoli: M. D'Auria, 1999, pp. 429–456.

Perilli 2011: Lorenzo Perilli, "Nuovi manoscritti del Glossario Ippocratico di Galeno e considerazioni stemmatiche. *Codex olim Mosquensis, codex Bodleianus Holkhamensis 92*", in Lorenzo Perilli, Christian Brockmann, Klaus-Dietrich Fischer, and Amneris Roselli (eds), *Officina Hippocratica. Beiträge zu Ehren von Anargyros Anastassiou und Dieter Irmer* (Beiträge zur Altertumskunde 289). Berlin and Boston, MA: De Gruyter, 2011, pp. 177–201.

Perrin 1988: Christophe Perrin, *La peau ou la représentation du corps malade: médecines antiques, médecine anatomo-clinique* (Thèse médecine) Nice: Université de Nice, 1988.

Petit 2006: Caroline Petit, "Les manuscrits de Modène et la tradition de l'*Introductio sive medicus* du Pseudo-Galien", in Véronique Boudon-Millot, Antonio Garzya, Jacques Jouanna, and Amneris Roselli (eds), *Ecdotica e ricezione dei testi medici greci. Atti del V Convegno Internazionale, Napoli, 1–2 ottobre 2004* (Collectanea 24). Napoli: M. D'Auria, 2006, pp. 167–185.

Pietrobelli 2010: Antoine Pietrobelli, "Variation autour du Thessalonicensis Vlatadon 14: un manuscrit copié au Xénon du Kral, peu avant la chute de Constantinople", *Revue des études byzantines* 68 (2010), pp. 95–126.

Pritchet 1975: Christopher Dixon Pritchet (ed.), *Iohannis Alexandrini Commentaria in sextum librum Hippocratis Epidemiarum recognovit et adnotatione critica instruxit*. Leiden: Brill, 1975.

Pritchet 1982: Christopher Dixon Pritchet (ed.), *Iohannis Alexandrini Commentaria in librum De sectis Galeni*. Recognovit et adnotatione critica instruxit. Leiden: E. J. Brill, 1982.

Raeder 1926: Ioannes Raeder (ed.), *Oribasii, Synopsis ad Eustathium; Libri ad Eunapium* (Corpus Medicorum Graecorum VI 3). Lipsiae et Berolini: B. G. Teubner, 1926.

Raeder 1928–1933: Ioannes Raeder (ed.), *Oribasii, Collectionum medicarum reliquiae*, 4 volumes (Corpus Medicorum Graecorum VI 1, 1–2; VI 2, 1–2). Lipsiae et Berolini: B. G. Teubner, 1928–1933.

Regling 1920: Kurt Regling, "Bruno Rappaport. Geb. den 4. November 1875, gest. den 20. Juli 1915", *Biographisches Jahrbuch für die Altertumswissenschaft* 40 (1920), pp. 76–83.

Rey 1993: Roselyne Rey, *Histoire de la douleur* (Histoire des sciences). Paris: La Découverte, 1993.

Richard 1948: Marcel Richard, *Répertoire des bibliothèques et des catalogues de nanuscrits grecs* (Publications de l'Institut de recherche et d'histoire des textes 1). Paris: Centre de documentation du Centre National de la Recherche Scientifique, 1948.

Richard 1958: Marcel Richard, *Répertoire des bibliothèques et des catalogues de manuscrits grecs*. Deuxième édition (Centre national de la recherche scientifique, Publications de l'Institut de recherche et d'histoire des textes 1). Paris: Centre national de la recherche scientifique, 1958.

Richard 1964: Marcel Richard, *Répertoire des bibliothèques et des catalogues de manuscrits grecs. Supplément I (1958–1963)* (Documents, études et répertoires publiés par l'Institut de recherche et d'histoire des textes 9). Paris: Éditions du Centre National de la Recherche Scientifique, 1964.

Rivier 1962: André Rivier, *Recherches sur la tradition manuscrite du traité hippocratique "De morbo sacro"* (Travaux publiés sous les auspices de la Société suisse des sciences morales 3). Berne: Francke, 1962.

Roselli 2009: Amneris Roselli, "Due manoscritti medici greci nelle biblioteche di Sofia", *Galenos* 3 (2009), pp. 177–180.

Sarton 1927–1948: George Sarton, *Introduction to the History of Science*, 3 volumes in five tomes. Baltimore: Williams & Wilkins, 1927–1948.

Sezgin 1970: Fuat Sezgin, *Geschichte des arabischen Schrifttums*, Band 3: *Medizin, Pharmazie, Zoologie, Tierheilkunde bis ca. 430 H.* Leiden: E.J.Brill, 1970.

Sezgin 1971: Fuat Sezgin, *Geschichte des arabischen Schrifttums*, Band 4: *Alchimie, Chemie, Botanik, Agrikultur bis ca. 430 H.* Leiden: E.J.Brill, 1971.

Sinkewicz 1990: Robert E. Sinkewicz, *Manuscript Listings for the Authors of Classical and Late Antiquity* (Greek Index Project Series 3). Toronto: Pontifical Institute of Mediaeval Studies, 1990.

Sinkewicz 1992: Robert E. Sinkewicz, *Manuscript Listings for the Authors of the Patristic and Byzantine Periods* (Greek Index Project Series 4). Toronto: Pontifical Institute of Mediaeval Studies, 1992.

Sinkewicz and Hayes 1989: Robert E. Sinkewicz and Walter H. Hayes, *Manuscript Listings for the Authored Works of the Palaeologan Period* (Greek Index Project Series 2). Toronto: Pontifical Institute of Mediaeval Studies, 1989.

Sonderkamp 1987: Joseph A. M. Sonderkamp, *Untersuchung zur Überlieferung der Schriften des Theophanes Chrysobalantes (sog. Theophanes Nonnus)* (Freie Universität Berlin, Byzantinisch-Neogriechisches Seminar, ΠΟΙΚΙΛΑ ΒΥΖΑΝΤΙΝΑ 7). Bonn: Dr. Rudolf Habelt, 1987.

Sprengel 1829: Kurt Sprengel (ed.), *Pedanii Dioscoridis Anazarbei De materia medica ad fidem codicum manuscriptorum, editionis aldinae principis usquequaque neglectae, et interpretum priscroum textum recnesuit, varias addidit lectiones, interpretationem emendavit, commentario illustravit*, Tomus I (Medicorum graecorum opoera quae exstant 1). Lipsiae: Cnobloch, 1829.

Thorndike and Kibre 1937: Lynn Thorndike, and Pearl Kibre, *A Catalogue of Incipits of Mediaeval Scientific Writings in Latin* (Mediaeval Academy of America, Publication 29). Cambridge, MA: Mediaeval Academy of America, 1937.

Thorndike and Kibre 1963: Lynn Thorndike, and Pearl Kibre, *A Catalogue of Incipits of Mediaeval Scientific Writings in Latin*. Revised and augmented edition (Mediaeval Academy of America, Publication 29). Cambridge, MA: Mediaeval Academy of America, 1963.

Touwaide 2009: Alain Touwaide, "Byzantine Medical Manuscripts. Towards a New Catalogue, with a Specimen for an Annotated Checklist of Manuscripts based on an Index of Diels' Catalogue", *Byzantion* 79 (2009), pp. 453–595.

Touwaide 2010: Alain Touwaide, "Codicology and Paleography", in Albrecht Classen (ed.), *Handbook of Medieval Studies. Terms, Methods, Trends*, 3 volumes. Berlin and New York, NY: Walter de Gruyter, 2010, vol. 1, pp. 266–329.

Touwaide 2016: Alain Touwaide, *A Census of Greek Medical Manuscripts. From Byzantium to the Renaissance* (Medicine in the Medieval Mediterranean 6). London and New York, NY: Routledge, 2016.

Touwaide 2018: Alain Touwaide, "Towards a Catalogue of Greek Medical Manuscripts", in Paola Degni, Paolo Eleuteri, and Marilena Maniaci (eds), *Greek Manuscript Cataloguing: Past, Present, and Future* (Bibliologia. Elementa ad librorum studia pertinentia 47). Turnhout: Brepols, 2018, pp. 111–118.

Tselikas 1995: Ἀγαμέμνων Τσελίκας, "Τὰ ἑλληνικὰ γιατροσόφια: μιὰ περιφρονημένη κατηγορία χειρογράφων", in Thanasis Diamantopoulos (ed.), Ιατρικά Βυζάντινα χειρόγραφα. Αθήνα: Δόμος, 1995, pp. 57–69.

Tselikas 2014: Ἀγαμέμνων Τσελίκας, "Δύο συναγωγὲς ἰατρικῶν λέξεων καὶ ἰατρικὲς συνταγὲς ἀπὸ τὸν ἰατροσοφικὸ κώδικα Παναγίου Τάφου 339 τοῦ Πατριαρχείου Ἱρουσολύμων", in *Εύκρατον-Πρακτικά Επιστημονικής Συνάντησης προς τιμήν του κ. Γεωργίου Ν. Αντονακοπούλου ομότιμου καθηγητού της Ιατρικής Σχολής του Πανεπιστημίου Θεσσαλίας. Λάρισσα 10 Μαΐου 2014, Αμφι-*

θέατρο Δημοσίας Κεντρικής Βιβλιοθήκης Λάρισσας «Κωνσταντίνος Κούμας». Λάρισσα: Δημοσίας Κεντρικής Βιβλιοθήκης Λάρισσας «Κωνσταντίνος Κούμας» – Ιατρική Σχολή Πανεπιστημίου Θεσσαλίας, 2014, pp. 107–176.

Tselikas and Ilioudis 1995: Ἀγαμέμνων Τσελίκας, Γιάννης Ἠλιούδης, *Νικολάου Ἱερόπαιδος ἐξ Ἀγράφων, Πραγματεία περὶ Φυσιολογίας καὶ Παθολογίας* (Βιβλιοθήκη Νεωτέρων Ἑλληνῶν Ἰατρῶν 1). Λάρισα: Πανεπιστήμιο Θεσσαλίας, Τμῆμα Ἰατρικῆς, 1995.

Tselikas and Ilioudis 1997: Ἀγαμέμνων Τσελίκας, Γιάννης Ἠλιούδης, *Νικολάου Ἱερόπαιδος ἐξ Ἀγράφων, Ἐκδόσεις μερικαὶ εἰς ἀρχάριον ἰατρόν* (Βιβλιοθήκη Νεωτέρων Ἑλληνῶν Ἰατρῶν 2). Λάρισα: Πανεπιστήμιο Θεσσαλίας, Τμῆμα Ἰατρικῆς, 1997.

Turyn 1932: Aleksander Turyn, *De Codicibus Pindaricis* (Polska Akademja Umiejętności: Archiwum Filologiczne 11). Cracoviae: Academia Polonae Litterarum, 1932.

Turyn 1943: Aleksander Turyn, *The Manuscript Tradition of the Tragedies of Aeschylus*. New York, NY: Polish Institute of Arts and Sciences in America, 1943.

Turyn 1952: Alexander Turyn, *Studies in the Manuscript Tradition of the Tragedies of Sophocles* (Illinois Studies in Language and Literature 36, 1–2.). Urbana, IL: University of Illinois Press, 1952.

Turyn 1957: Alexander Turyn, *The Byzantine Manuscript Tradition of the Tragedies of Euripides* (Illinois Studies in Language and Literature 43). Urbana, IL: University of Illinois Press, 1957.

Ullmann 1970: Manfred Ullmann, *Die Medizin im Islam* (Handbuch der Orientalistik, Erste Abteilung: Der nahe und der mittlere Osten, Ergänzungsband VI, 1. Abschnitt). Leiden and Köln: Brill, 1970.

Verner 1966: Mathilde Verner "Johann Albert Fabricius, Eighteenth-Century Scholar and Bibliographer", *The Papers of the Bibliographical Society of America* 60 (3) (1966), pp. 281–326.

Voigts and Kurtz 2004: Linda Ersham Voigts, and Patricia Deery Kurtz, *Electronic Thorndike Kibre (eTK) and Electronic Voigts Kurtz (eVK)*. CD Rom publication, release 20 August 2004.

Vollmer 1916: Fridericus Vollmer, *Quinti Sereni Liber medicinalis*. Edidit – (Corpus Medicorum Latinorum II 3). Lipsiae et Berolini: B. G. Teubner, 1916.

Wellmann 1908: Max Wellmann (ed.), *Philumeni de venenatis animalibus eorumque remediis ex codice vaticano* primum edidit (Corpus Medicorum Graecorum X 1, 1). Lipsiae et Berolini: B. G. Teubner, 1908.

Wenkebach 1934: Ernst Wenkebach (ed.), *Galeni, In Hippocratis epidemiarum librum I commentarii III*; Franz Pfarr (Germ. transl.), *Galeni, In Hippocratis epidemiarum librum II commentarii V* (Corpus Medicorum Graecorum V 10, 1). Lipsiae et Berolini: B. G. Teubner, 1934.

Wenkebach 1936: Ernst Wenkebach (ed.), *Galeni, In Hippocratis epidemiarum librum IIII commentarii III* (Corpus Medicorum Graecorum V 10, 2. 1). Lipsiae et Berolini: B. G. Teubner, 1936.

Wilson 1987: Nigel G. Wilson, "Aspects of the Transmission of Galen", in Guglielmo Cavallo (ed.), *Le strade del testo* (Studi e commenti 5). Bari: Adriatica Editrice, 1987, pp. 45–64.

Zipser 2009: Barbara Zipser (ed.), *John the Physician's Therapeutics. A Medical Handbook in Vernacular Greek* (Studies in Ancient Medicine 37). Leiden: Brill, 2009.

Acknowledgements

This work is the result of decades of intensive activity in libraries, research centers, universities, and other institutions throughout the world, which have all provided resources, access to collections, expertise and guidance and, most simply, a home. I am pleased to thank all of them and their staff, even though I cannot enumerate them here. In very recent years, the work has benefitted from the active support of De Gruyter, particularly the Senior Editor for Classical Studies Dr. Serena Pirrotta and her team, especially Marco Acquafredda, and De Gruyter computer and technical units in the persons of Anne Hiller and Florian Ruppenstein who have provided much needed assistance. Going slightly back in time, Patricia Kellogg has been an efficient research assistant and Cheyenne Moore has checked the accuracy of my index of Diels against the original. Since its foundation in 2007 the *Institute for the Preservation of Medical Traditions* has hosted the programme. In the very last phase, Marisa Gomez has checked with great linguistic talent the correctness of the introduction to the several parts of the work. More than anyone else, Emanuela Appetiti has accompanied me through multiple peregrinations of all kinds of which this work may give only an imperfect idea. I cannot conclude without remembering Joseph A. M. Sonderkamp with whom I discussed the project of a *New Diels* and a catalogue of Greek medical manuscripts as early as 1983 in Berlin and then in 1987 at Louvain-la-Neuve. We had defined a cooperative programme and had started implementing it when the sinister *Moira* decided shortly after that we would not fully realize it in collaboration.

Index of Manuscripts
Diels' Location and Shelfmark

Notes for consultation

This index lists all the manuscripts with Hippocratic and related texts mentioned in Diels. The identifications exactly reproduce the data provided in Diels, the majority of which comprise the following three or four components: city (German form), library (mostly in the original language, often in an abbreviated form, and in their form as in Diels' time), collection (when appropriate), and one or more shelfmarks or references to an earlier work. In some cases, the name of the library is not explicitly mentioned; it can be identified through the list of catalogues in Diels' bibliography. The index references the page number(s) where each item appears in the present volume.

This index is preceded by a **Finding Aid** which lists the city, library and collection names in alphabetical order with reference to the present index, and two lists: one with the names as in Diels (sometimes including transliteration into the Latin alphabet for Greek names) and the other with their current standard English form.

Finding Aid

City and Library names

1. Names according to Diels

Amsterdam, Universitätsbibliothek: xli
Antwerpen, Stadtbibliothek: xli
Athen: xli
  Βιβλ. τῆς Βουλῆς: xli
  Nationalbibl.: xli
Athos: xli
  Βιβλ. Μον. Διονυσίου: xli
  Βιβλ. Μον. Δοχειαρίου: xli
  Βιβλ. Μον. Ἐσφιγμένου: xli
  Βιβλ. Μον. Ἰβήρων: xli
  Βιβλ. Μον. Παντελεήμονος: xlii
  Βιβλ. Μον. Ξηροποταμοῦ: xlii

Berlin, Königl. Bibl.: xlii
    4°/qu.: xlii
    fol.: xlii
    Phillipps.: xlii
Bern, Stadtbibliothek: xlii
Bologna, Bibl. Universitaria: xlii
Brüssel, Königl. Bibl.: xliii

Cambridge: xliii
  [Ashmol.]: xliii
  Caius Coll.: xliii
  Cantabrig. Bibl. Univ.: xliii
Chalke, Βιβλ. μον. Θεοτόκου: xliii

Erlangen, Universitätsbibliothek: xliii
Escurial: xliii

Florenz: xliv
  Bibl. Marucell.: xliv
  Bibl. Mediceo Laurentiana: xliv
    Conv. soppr.: xliv
    Laurent. App.: xliv
    Laurent. plut.: xliv
  Bibl. Magliabech./bibl. naz.: xliv
  Bibl. Riccardiana: xlv

Göttingen, Univ.-Bibl.: xlv
  Hist. nat.: xlv
  Philol.: xlv

Heidelberg, Bibl. Univ.: xlv
Holkham, Bibl. des Gr. Leicester: xlv

Jerusalem: xlv
  Bibl. d. hl. Grabes: xlv
  Bibl. Mar-Saba: xlv
  Bibl. patriarch.: xlv

Karlsruhe, Großherzogl. Hof. u.
  Landesbibliothek: xlv
Kopenhagen, Königl. Bibliothek: xlvi

Leipzig, Universitätsbibliothek: xlvi
Lesbos, Βιβλ. τῆς τοῦ Λειμῶνος Μονῆς: xlvi
Leyden, Universitätsbibliothek: xlvi
  B. P.: xlvi
  Scal.: xlvi
  Voss.: xlvi
    Voss. 4°: xlvi
    Voss. 8°: xlvi
    Voss. fol.: xlvi
    Voss. Miscell.: xlvi
  Vulc.: xlvi
London: xlvi
  British Museum: xlvi
    Addit.: xlvi
    Arundel.: xlvi
    Harleian.: xlvi
    Regius: xlvii
    Stowe: xlvii
  Medical Society: xlvii

Madrid, Nationalbibliothek: xlvii

Mailand: xlvii
Bibl. Ambrosiana: xlvii
Bibl. Trivulziana: xlviii
Modena, Bibl. Estense: xlviii
Moskau, Synodialbibl.: xlviii
München, Hof- und Staatsbibliothek: xlviii

Neapel: xlviii
Biblioteca Borbonica: xlviii
Bibl. dei Gerolamini: xlix
Bibl. di S. Giovanni di Carbonara: xlix
Bibl. Oratoriana: xlix

Oxford: xlix
Bibl. Aedis Christi: xlix
Bibl. Bodleiana: xlix
Auct.: xlix
Baroccian.: xlix
Canonician.: xlix
Clarkian.: xlix
Ger. Langbainii Advers.: xlix
Miscell.: xlix
Orvillian: xlix
Roe: l

Padua: l
Bibl. Canonicor. Lateran.: l
Bibl. S. Joannis in Viridario: l
Palermo, Biblioteca nazionale: l
Paris: l
Bibl. de Paris: l
Bibl. Facult. Med.: l
Bibl. Nationale: l
Coislin.: l
Parisin.: l
Suppl.: liv
Bibl. Regia: l
Pistoja, Biblioteca Fabroniana: liv

Rom: liv
Bibl. Angelica: liv
Bibl. Barberin.: liv
Bibl. Corsiniana: liv
Bibl. Vallicellana: lv
Bibl. Vaticana: lv
Ottobon.: lv
Palat.: lv
Reg. Suec.: lv
Urbin.: lv
Vatic.: lv

Sens, Bibl. communale: lvi

Tübingen, Univ.-Bibl.: lvi
Turin, Bibl. Nazionale (Universitaria): lvi

Upsala, Upsal. bibl. acad.: lvii

Venedig: lvii
Bibl. Nazionale Marciana: lvii
appendix graeca: lvii
graeci: lvii
Bibl. S. Anton.: lvii

Wien: lviii
Bibl. Colleg. S. J. Rossia: lviii
Gollob Privatbesitz: lviii
Hofbibliothek: lviii
histor.: lviii
lat.: lviii
med.: lviii
phil.: lix
philos. et philol.: lix
theol.: lix
Wolfenbüttel, Bibl. Guelf. August.: lix
August.: lix
Guelferb.: lix

Zaragoza, Bibl. d. Cat. d. Pil.: lix
Zürich, Stadtbibliothek: lix

2. Standard English names

Amsterdam, University Library: xli
Antwerp, City Library: xli
Athens: xli
  National Library: xli
  Parliament Library: xli
Athos (Mount –): xli
  Dionysiou Monastery: xli
  Dochiariou Monastery: xli
  Esfigmenou Monastery: xli
  Iviron Monastery: xli
  Panteleimonos Monastery: xlii
  Xiropotamou Monastery: xlii

Berlin, Royal Library: xlii
  4°/qu: xlii
  fol.: xlii
  Phillipps.: xlii
Bern, City Library: xlii
Bologna, University Library: xlii
Brussels, Royal Library: xliii

Cambridge: xliii
  [Ashmol.]: xliii
  Caius College: xliii
  University Library: xliii
Chalki, Library of the Theotokou Monastery: xliii
Copenhagen, Royal Library: xlvi

Erlangen, University Library: xliii
Escorial (San Lorenzo de El –), Monastery Library: xliii

Florence: xliv
  Marucelliana Library: xliv
  Medicea Laurenziana Library: xliv
    Conv. soppr.: xliv
    Laurent. App.: xliv
    Laurent. plut.: xliv
  National Library: xliv
  Riccardiana Library: xlv

Göttingen, University Library: xlv
  Hist. nat.: xlv
  Philol.: xlv

Heidelberg, University Library: xlv
Hokham, Library of the Earl of Leicester: xlv

Jerusalem: xlv
  Library of the Holy Sepulchre: xlv
  Mar-Sabba Library: xlv
  Patriarchal Library: xlv

Karlsruhe, Library of Grand Duchy Court and State: xlv

Leipzig, University Library: xlvi
Lesvos, Library of the Limonos Monastery: xlvi
Leiden, University Library: xlvi
  B. P.: xlvi
  Scal.: xlvi
  Voss.: xlvi
    Voss. 4°: xlvi
    Voss. 8°: xlvi
    Voss. fol.: xlvi
    Voss. Miscell.: xlvi
  Vulc.: xlvi
London: xlvi
  British Museum: xlvi
    Addit.: xlvi
    Arundel.: xlvi
    Harleian.: xlvi
    Regius: xlvii
    Stowe: xlvii
  Medical Society: xlvii

Madrid, National Library: xlvii
Milan: xlvii
  Ambrosiana Library: xlvii
  Trivulziana Library: xlviii
Modena, Estense Library: xlviii
Moscow, Synodial Library: xlviii
Munich, Court and State Library: xlviii

Naples: xlviii
  Girolamini Library: xlix
  Oratory Library: xlix
  Royal Borbonica Library: xlviii
  St. John Library at Carbonara: xlix

Oxford: xlix
Bodleian Library: xlix
Auct.: xlix
Baroccian.: xlix
Canonician.: xlix
Clarkian.: xlix
Ger. Langbainii Advers.: xlix
Miscell.: xlix
Orvillian: xlix
Roe: l
Christ Churchi Library: xlix

Padua: l
Library of Canons Regular of the Lateran: l
St. John in Viridario Library: l
Palermo, National Library: l
Paris: l
Medical School Library: l
National Library: l
Coislin.: l
Parisin.: l
Suppl.: liv
Paris Library: l
Royal Library: l
Pistoia, Fabroniana Library: liv

Rome: liv
Angelica Library: liv
Barberiniana Library: liv
Corsiniana Library: liv
Vallicelliana Library: lv
Vatican Library: lv
Ottobon.: lv
Palat.: lv
Reg. Suec.: lv
Urbin.: lv
Vatic.: lv

Sens, Municipal Library: lvi

Tübingen, University Libray: lvi
Turin, National Library (University Library): lvi

Uppsala, Library of the Academy: lvii

Venice: lvii
National Library: lvii
appendix graeca: lvii
graeci: lvii
St Antonio Library: lvii
Vienna: lviii
Court Library: lviii
histor.: lviii
lat.: lviii
med.: lviii
phil.: lix
philos. et philol.: lix
theol.: lix
Private Collection Eduard Gollob: lviii
Rossia Library of Jesuit Company College: lviii

Wolfenbüttel, August Guelph's Library: lix
August.: lix
Guelferb.: lix

Zaragoza, Cathedral Library: lix
Zürich, City Library: lix

Index of Manuscripts

[Amsterdam, Universitäts-Bibliothek]
[?]: 5

Antwerpen, Stadtbibliothek
426: 5

Athen, Βιβλ. τῆς Βουλῆς
39: 5
68: 5

Athen, Nationalbibl.
1477: 6
1486: 6
1488: 6
1498: 6
1500: 6
1504: 6

Athos, Βιβλ. Μον. Διονυσίου
3701.167: 6
3758.224: 6

Athos, Βιβλ. Μον. Δοχειαρίου
2917.243: 7

Athos, Βιβλ. Μον. Ἐσφιγμένου
2323.310: 7
2330.317: 7

Athos, Βιβλ. Μον. Ἰβήρων
4212.92: 7
4271.151: 7
4294.174: 8
4302.182: 8
4304.184: 8
4309.189: 8
4310.190: 8

4330.310: 8
4338.218: 8
4340.220: 8
4463.343: 9
4501.381: 9
4655.535: 9
4671.551: 9
5034.914: 9

Athos, Βιβλ. Μον. Παντελεήμονος
5769.262: 9
5796.289: 9
6342.835: 10

Athos, Βιβλ. Μον. Ξηροποτάμου
2432.99: 10

Berlin, Königl. Bibl.
fol. 39 (275): 10
qu. 5 (304): 10
Phillipps.
1462: 10
1487: 11
1524 (ol. Meerm. 214): 11
1525 (ol. Meerm. 215): 11
1527 (ol. Meerm. 217): 11
1529 (ol. Meerm. 220): 11
1532 (ol. Meerman. 225): 11
1533: 11
1537 (ol. Meerman. 233): 12
1538 (ol. Meerm. 233): 12
1566 (ol. Meerm. 269): 12
1583: 12

Bern, Stadtbibliothek
579: 12

Bologna, Bibl. Universitaria
3232: 12
3563: 12
3632: 12

3633: 13
3636: 13

Brüssel, Königl. Bibl.
1871–77: 13
11345–48: 13

[Cambridge, Ashmol.]
[7751]: 13

Cambridge, Caius Coll.
50: 14
76: 14
355: 15
[949]: 15

Cambridge, Cantabrig. Bibl. Univ.
2049 (Kk V 7): 15
[2329]: 15
L l IV 12: 15
L. L. 5, 4: 15

Chalke, Βιβλ. μον. Θεοτόκου
82: 16

Erlangen, Universitätsbibliothek
Bibl. Univ. 90: 16

Escurial, Scorial
Σ. II. 5: 16
Σ. II. 10: 16
Σ. II. 11: 16
T. II. 12: 17
T. II. 14: 17
Y. III. 10: 17
Υ III 17: 17
Υ. III. 17: 17
y. I. 8: 17
y. I. 9 : 17
y. III. 16: 17
Φ. I. 10: 18

Φ. III. 7: 18
Φ. III. 11: 18
Φ. III. 12: 18
Ψ. III. 17: 18

Florenz, Bibl. Marucell.
A 109: 18

Florenz, Bibl. Mediceo Laurentiana
Conv. soppr.
153: 19
Laurent
[plut. 25, ?]: 19
[plut. 25, ?]: 19
plut. 59, 14: 19
plut. 71, 1: 19
plut. 74, 1: 19
plut. 74, 3: 21
plut. 74, 7: 21
plut. 74, 8: 21
plut. 74, 10: 21
plut. 74, 11: 21
[plut. 74, 12]: 22
plut. 74, 13: 22
plut. 74, 21: 22
plut. 74, 25: 22
plut. 74, 31: 22
plut. 75, 3: 22
plut. 75, 5: 22
plut. 75, 10: 23
[plut. 75, 10]: 23
plut. 75, 19: 23
plut. 75, 21: 23
plut. 75, 22: 23
Laurent. App.
2: 23

Florenz, Magliabech.
1: 24

Florenz, bibl. naz. [Magliabecchiana]
II.III.428: 24

Florenz, Bibl. Riccardiana
17 (K I 24): 24
41 (K II 2): 24
44 (K II 5): 24

Göttingen, Univ.-Bibl.
Hist. nat.
3: 25
4: 25
5: 25
Philol.
2: 25
21: 25

Heidelberg, Bibl. Univ.
132: 25
155: 26
398: 26

Holkham, Bibl. des Gr. Leicester
282: 26
293: 27

Jerusalem, Bibl. d. hl. Grabes
189: 27

Jerusalem, Bibl. Mar-Saba
432: 27
481: 27
498: 28

Jerusalem, Bibl. patriarch.
102: 28
148: 28
463: 28

Karlsruhe, Großherzogl. Hof. u. Landesbibliothek
449: 28

Kopenhagen, Königl. Bibliothek
Hauniens. ant. fund. reg.
224: 29

Leipzig, Universitätsbibliothek
56: 30
59: 30
61: 31
64: 31

Lesbos, Βιβλ. τῆς τοῦ Λειμῶνος Μονῆς
175: 31

Leyden, Universitäts-Bibliothek
B. P.
670: 31
Scalig.
71: 31
Voss. 4°
38: 32
50: 32
Voss. 8°
7: 32
Voss. fol.
10: 32
Voss. Miscell.
1 pars 13: 33
Vulc.
56: 33
108 pars 15: 33

London, British Museum
Addit./Addit. (Brit. Mus.)
6898: 33
28, 830: 33
34,060: 34
Arundel./Arundelian.
538: 34
Harleian.
5611: 34
5626: 34

5635: 34
6295: 34
6301: 35
Regius
16. C. XVI: 35
Stowe
1073: 35

London, Medical Society
AA a 1 = Xa 32: 35
HHi 17 = We 30: 35
HH i 21. 22 = We 28. 29: 35

Madrid, Nationalbibliothek
4557 (N 119): 36
4634 (olim N 112): 36

Mailand, Bibl. Ambrosiana
A 45 Sup.: 36
A 95 Sup.: 36
A 110 Sup.: 36
A 156 Sup.: 36
B 72 Sup.: 37
B 108 Sup.: 37
B 113 Sup.: 37
B 126 Sup.: 37
C 4 Sup.: 37
C 85 Sup.: 38
C 118 Sup.: 38
C 119 Sup.: 38
F 23 Sup.: 38
L 30 Sup.: 39
L 110 Sup.: 39
P 90 Sup.: 39
Q 3 Sup.: 40
Q 13 Sup.: 40
S 19 Sup.: 40
T 19 Sup.: 40
A 27 Inf. : 40
H 2 Inf.: 40
S.Q.E. VIII 13: 40

S.Q.T. VIII 9: 40

Mailand, Bibl. Trivulziana
685: 41

Modena, Bibl. Estense
54 (III B 2): 41
61 (III B 9): 41
85 (III C 6): 41
115 (II D 16): 41
191: 42
211 (III G 7): 42
213 (III G 9): 42
218 (II H 3): 42
220 (II H 5): 42
227 (II H 12): 42
233 (III H 5): 43
237 (III G 18): 43
240 (III F 17): 43

Moskau, Synodialbibl.
[?]: 44
439: 44
465: 44
466: 44

München, Hof- und Staatsbibliothek
graec.
71: 45
72: 46
227: 46
231: 47
276: 47
287: 47
469: 47
494: 47
525: 47

Neapel, Biblioteca Borbonica
III C 2 (260): 48
91 (II C 33): 48

187 (II F 30): 48

Neapel, Bibl. dei Gerolamini
XXII.1: 48

Neapel, Bibl. di S. Giovanni di Carbonara
15: 49
27: 49

Neapel, Bibl. Oratoriana
152: 49

Oxford, Bibl. Aedis Christi
34: 49

Oxford, Bibl. Bodleiana
Auct.
F. Inf. II 3: 49
T II 3: 50
T II 10: 50
Baroccian.
10: 50
51: 50
76: 50
88: 50
131: 50
150: 50
204: 51
224: 52
Canonician.
1: 52
Clarkian.
16 (18378): 52
Ger. Langbainii Advers.
2: 52
Miscell.
130: 53
132: 53
210: 53
d'Orvillian.
X 1. 1. 3: 53

X 1. 4. 29: 53
Roe.
14 (260): 53
14 (Bodl. 260): 54
XIV (260): 54

[Padua, Bibl. Canonicor. Lateranens.]
[–]: 54

Padua, Bibl. S. Joannis in Viridario
ad dextr. plut. XVII: 54

Palermo, Biblioteca nazionale
XIII C 3: 55

[Paris, Bib.Regia/B. R.]
[120 ap. Montf. II 902]: 55

Paris, Bibl. de Paris
4: 55

Paris, Bibl. Facult. Med. / Bibl. Facult. Medic. / Faculté de Méd.
–: 56
14: 55, 56

Paris, Bibl. Nationale
Coislin.
163: 56
321: 56
[321 (?)]: 56
335: 56
[335]: 57
Parisin.
36: 57 (36), 88 ([3170 (?)])
396: 57
985: 57
1297: 57
1327: 57
[1444 (?)]: 57, 60–70 (2140–2146), 78 (2255)
1630: 58
[1667 (?)]: 58, 59 (1884)

1760: 58
[1848 ?]: 58, 59 (1884)
1849: 58
1868: 58
1883: 59
1884: 58 ([1667 (?)], [1848 ?]), 59 (1884), ([1884]), ([1884 (?)]), ([1885]), ([1885 (?)])
[1884]: 59
[1884 (?)]: 59
[1885]: 59
[1885 (?)]: 59
1995: 60
[2030]: 60 ([2030]), 83 (2330)
2047: 60
2091: 60
2140: 57 ([1444 (?)]), 60
[2140]: 60 (2140), 61 ([2140])
2141: 57 ([1444 (?)]), 61, 63 ([2141])
[2141]: 61 (2141), 63 ([2141])
2142: 57 ([1444 (?)]), 63 (2142), 64 ([2142]), 75 ([2242 (?)])
[2142]: 63 (2142), 64 ([2142]), 75 ([2242 (?)])
2143: 57 ([1444 (?)]), 64 (2143), 66 ([2143]),([2143 (?)]), 71 ([2148])
[2143]: 64 (2143), 66 ([2143])
[2143 (?)]: 64 (2143), 66 ([2143 (?)])
2144: 57 ([1444 (?)]), 66 (2144), 67 ([2144]), 72 ([2154])
[2144]: 66 (2144), 67 ([2144])
2145: 57 ([1444 (?)]), 68 (2145), 69 ([2145]), 72 ([2154]), 85 (2545 [? = 2145 ? cf. Kühn I. 1]), ([2545 (?) = 2145 ?]), ([2545 (? = 2145 ?)])
[2145]: 68 (2145), 69 ([2145])
2146: 57 ([1444 (?)]), 69 (2146), 70 ([2146]), ([2146 (?)], 86 ([2546 (? = 2146?)])
[2146]: 69 (2146), 70 ([2146])
[2146 (?)]: 60 (2140), 69 (2146), 70 ([2146 (?)])
2147: 70 (2147), ([2147])
[2147]: 70 (2147), ([2147])
[2147 (?)]: 70 (2147), 71 ([2147 (?)])
[2148]: 64 (2143), 71 ([2148])
2149: 71 (2149), 72 (2149 [?])
2149 (?): 71 (2149), 72 (2149 [?])
2150: 72
2151: 72

[2154]: 66 (2144), 68 (2145), 72 ([2154])
2155: 72
2161: 72
2165: 72
2166: 72
2168: 73
2174: 73
2177: 73
2178: 73
2219: 73
2222: 73
2223: 74
2224: 74
2228: 74 (2228), 87 ([2828 (? = 2228?)])
2229: 74 (2229), [2229 (?)])
[2229 (?)]: 74 (2229), ([2229 (?)])
[2232]: 75 ([2232]), 83 (2332)
2240: 75 (2240), 87 ([2269 (?)])
[2242 (?)]: 63 (2142), 75 ([2242 (?)])
2247: 75 (2247), ([2247])
[2247]: 75 (2247), ([2247])
2248: 75 (2248), 76 ([2248])
[2248]: 75 (2248), 76 ([2248])
[2250]: 76 ([2250]), 80 (2256), (2258), (2259)
2253: 76 (2253), ([2253]), 114 ([Venedig. Bibl. S. Anton.])
[2253]: 76 (2253), ([2253])
2254: 76 (2254), 80 ([2257 (?)])
[2254]: 77 ([2254]), 78 (2255)
[2254 (?)]: 77 ([2254 (?)]), 78 (2255)
2255: 57 ([1444 (?)]),77 ([2254]), ([2254 (?)]), 78 (2255), 79 ([2255]), ([2255 (?)]
[2255]: 78 (2255), 79 ([2255])
[2255 (?)]: 78 (2255), 79 ([2255 (?)])
2256: 76 ([2250]), 80 (2256), 81 ([2266 9?]))
2257: 80 (2257), 87 ([3140 (?)])
[2257 (?)]: 76 (2254), 80 ([2257 (?)])
2258: 76 ([2250]), 80 (2258)
2259: 76 ([2250]), 80 (2258)
2260: 80 (2260)
2266: 80 (2266), 81 ([2266 (?)])
[2266 (?)]:80 (2266), 81 ([2266 (?)])
2268: 81

2269: 81 (2269), ([2269])
[2269]: 81 (2269), ([2269])
2276: 81
2278: 81
2287: 82
2294: 82
2295: 82
2296: 82
2301: 82 (2301) ([2301 (?)])
[2301 (?)]: 82 (2301) ([2301 (?)])
2304: 82
2308: 82
2315: 82
2316: 83
2317: 83
2320: 83
2330: 60 ([2030]), 83 (2330)
2332: 75 ([2232]), 83 (2332), ([2332])
[2332]: 83 (2332), ([2332])
2419: 84
2510: 85
2545 (? = 2145 ? cf. Kühn l.1): 68 (2145), 85 (2545 [? = 2145 ? cf. Kühn l.1])
[2545 (?) = 2145 ?]: 68 (2145), 85 ([2545 (?) = 2145 ?])
[2545 (? = 2145 ?)]: 68 (2145), 85 ([2545 (? = 2145 ?)])
[2546 (? = 2146 ?)]: 69 (2146), 86 ([2546 (? = 2146 ?)])
2596: 86
2614: 86
2615: 86
2651: 86
2652: 86
2671: 86 (2671), 87 ([2671 (?)])
[2671 (?)]: 86 (2671), 87 ([2671 (?)])
[2699 (?)]: 75 (2240), 87 ([2269 (?)])
2755: 87
[2828 (? = 2228 ?)]: 74 (2228), 87 ([2828 (? = 2228?)])
2847: 87
2894: 87
3047: 87
3050: 87
3052: 87
[3140 (?)]: 80 (2257), 87 ([3140 (?)])

[3170 (?)]: 57 (36), 88 ([3170 (?)])
Suppl. gr.
2: 88
64: 88
165: 88
205: 88
270: 88
352: 88
446: 88
447: 89 (447), 118 (Wien, Hofbibliothek, Vindob. med. 34)
496: 89
608: 89
637: 89 (637), (675)
675: 89 (637), (675)
682: 89
684: 89
688: 90
728 (Minas IZ): 90 (728 [Minas IZ]), (1254)
754 (Minas): 90 (754 [Minas]), (1254)
1194: 90
1254: 90 (728 [Minas IZ]), (754 [Minas]), (1254)

Pistoja, Biblioteca Fabroniana
141 (308): 90

Rom, Bibl. Angelica
4 (C.4.16): 91
80 (C.1. 11): 91

Rom, Bibl. Barberin.
I 5: 91
I 11 (= 136): 91 (I 11), 92 (136 [= I 11])
I 127: 91 (I 127), 92 (276)
III 63 (= 245): 92
136 (= I 11): 91 (I 11), 92 (136 [= I 11])
276: 91 (I 127), 92 (276)

Rom, Bibl. Corsiniana (= Acc. d. Lincei)
1410 (36. E. 26): 92

Rom, Bibl. Vallicellana
- 78 (F 9): 92
- 1106 (F 83): 93

Rom, Bibl. Vaticana
- Ottobon.
  - 150: 93
  - 157 A: 93
  - 157 B: 93
  - 192: 93
- Palat.
  - 126: 93
  - 128: 93
  - 129: 93
  - 132: 94
  - 143: 94
  - 155: 94
  - 157: 94
  - 173: 94 (Palat. 173), 96 (Reg. Suec. 173)
  - 192: 94
  - 199: 95
  - 278: 95
  - 279: 95
  - 297: 96
  - 363: 96
  - 385: 96
  - 398: 96
  - 400: 96
  - 428: 96
- Reg. Suec.
  - 173: 94 (Palat. 173), 96 (Reg. Suec. 173)
  - 175: 97
  - 181: 97
  - 182: 97
- Urbin.
  - 64: 97
  - 65: 98
  - 67: 98
  - 68: 98
- Vatic.
  - [216]: 100 ([Vatic. 216]), 102 (Vatic. 278)

276: 100
277: 101
278: 100 ([Vatic. 216]), 102 (Vatic. 278)
279: 103
280: 104
283: 104
285: 104
293: 104
294: 104
690: 104
876: 104
1062: 104
1063: 104
1065: 105
1066: 105
1095: 105
1133 (1134 Kl.): 105
1276: 105
1309: 105
1354: 105
1467: 105
1759: 105
1858: 105
1879: 106
2154: 106
2238: 106
2254: 106
2304 [olim 2217]: 106

Sens, Bibl. communale
Miscell. 187: 106

Tübingen, Univ.-Bibl.
23: 106
37: 107

Turin, Bibl. Nazionale (Universitaria)
156 b II 10: 107
177 b II 31: 107
179 b II 33: 107 (179 b II 33), (B V 33 [179 b II 33])
287 c I 42: 107 (287 c I 42), 108 (C VI 3 [287 c I 42])

B V 33 (179 b II 33): 107 (179 b II 33), (B V 33 [179 b II 33])
C VI 3 (287 c I 42): 107 (287 c I 42), 108 (C VI 3 [287 c I 42])
C VI 21 (b VI 18): 108

Upsala, Upsal. bibl. acad.
8 (e don. Jo. Gabr. Sparfwenf. 49): 108
34: 108

Venedig, Bibl. Nazionale Marciana
graeci
[–]: 108 ([Marcian.]), 109 (graecus 269)
[–]: 109 ([Marcian.]), (graecus 269)
[?]: 109 ([Marcian. ?]), (graecus 269)
[ap. Montfaucon, I 472]: 109 ([ap. Montfaucon, I 472]), 111 (graecus 283)
269: 108 ([Marcian.]), 109 ([Marcian.]), ([Marcian. ?]), (graecus 269)
277: 110
278: 110
279: 111
281: 111
282: 111
283: 109 ([ap. Montfaucon, I 472]), 111 (graecus 283)
285: 111
296: 112
609: 112
appendix graeca
V, 4: 112
V, 5: 112
V, 9: 112
V, 10: 113
V, 13: 113
V, 14: 113 (V, 14), (V, 14 [olim Nanian. 248])
V, 14 (olim Nanian. 248): 113 (V, 14), (V, 14 [olim Nanian. 248])
V, 15: 113
V, 16: 113
V, 19: 114

[Venedig], [Bibl. S. Anton.]
–: 114 ([Venedig, Bibl. S. Anton.]), 115 (Wien, Hofbibliothek, histor. 130)
–: 76 (Paris, graecus 2253), 114 ([Venedig, Bibl. S. Anton.]),

Wien, Bibl. Colleg. S. J. Rossianus
XI.167: 114

Wien, Gollob Privatbesitz
Vindob.: 115

Wien, Hofbibliothek
[Lamb. VI 85]: 115 ([Lamb. VI 85]), 116 ((Wien, Hofbibliothek, med. 4)
[ap. Nessel. P. III]: 115
69 B 101: 115
[179]: 115
hist./histor.
130: 114 ([Venedig, Bibl. S. Anton.]), 115 (Wien, Hofbibliothek, histor. 130)
lat.
4772 (tab. Cod. III 382): 116
med.
4: 115 ([Lamb. VI 85]), 116 ((Wien, Hofbibliothek, med. 4)
8: 116 (med. 8), (med. [8])
[8]: 116 (med. 8), (med. [8])
13: 116 (med. 13)
14: 116 (med. 14)
[15]: 117 (med. [15])
16: 117 (med. 16), (med. 16 [ol. 35])
16 (ol. 35): 117 (med. 16), (med. 16 [ol. 35])
24: 117 (med. 24)
28: 117 (med. 28), ([med. 28])
[28 (?)]: 117 (med. 28), ([med. 28 (?)])
31: 118 (med. 31)
32: 118 (med. 32)
34: 118 (med. 34)
38 ^{c}: 118 (med. 38 ^{c})
40: 118 (med. 40)
41: 118 (med. 41), 119 ([med. 41])
[41]: 118 (med. 41), 119 ([med. 41])
43: 119 (med. 43)
44: 119 (med. 44)
47: 119 (med. 47)
48: 119 (med. 48)
49: 119 (med. 49)
52: 119 (med. 52)
53: 120 (med. 53), ([med. 53])

[53]: 120 (med. 53), ([med. 53])
phil.
74: 120 (phil. 74)
82: 120 (phil. 82)
178: 120 (phil. 178)
179: 120 (phil. 179), 121 (philos. et philol. 179)
192: 121 (phil. 192)
219 : 121 (phil. 219)
philos. et philol.
179: 120 (phil. 179), 121 (philos. et philol. 179)
theol.
293: 121 (theol. 293)

Wolfenbüttel, Bibl. Guelf. August./Bibl. Guelf.
[Augustiani 18, 1]: 121
Guelferbyt. 3132 (18.1 Aug. 4°): 121

Zaragoza, Bibl. d. Cat. d. Pil.
1115 (olim 1427): 121

Zürich, Stadtbibliothek
C 136: 122

Index of Manuscripts
Current location and shelfmark

Notes for consultation

This index lists all the Greek manuscripts mentioned in Diels that have been preserved and identified since[1]. Their designation comprises their current location and shelfmark, with the following three or four components: city, library, collection (when appropriate), and shelfmark. All names are in the original language and alphabet, followed by their transliteration into Latin alphabet and translation into English for those in the original Russian and Armenian alphabet and form. Each entry of the index references the page number(s) in this volume where the manuscripts appear.

Since the manuscripts contained in the catalogue in this volume are identified as they are in Diels, consultation of the catalogue on the basis of this index might be problematic because current designations do not always match Diels' designations. In Diels, indeed, cities are identified by their German names, libraries are often designated in an abbreviated form, collection names are abbreviated or may not reflect actual names, and shelfmarks are sometimes insufficient or inexact, or even include earlier ones. Additionally, changes have occurred since Diels' time in the location of some collections and several manuscripts, in the names of some libraries and, also, in the shelfmarks (and even in the shelfmark system) of several libraries. Diels' identifiers are reproduced between parentheses after the page number referring to the mention(s) of the manuscripts in the catalogue contained in this volume. In the catalogue itself, both designations of manuscripts are included when appropriate, followed by the current one (as listed in the present index).

This index is preceded by a **Finding Aid** which provides the current city, library, and collection names in alphabetical order with reference to the present index. All names are in the original language and alphabet.

---

1 This index does not include the manuscripts that have been lost or destroyed (*in toto* or *in parte*) since (e.g. some items from Dresden or Torino), the manuscripts that cannot be exactly identified on the basis of Diels' information, the papyri, and the Latin and Arabic manuscripts included among the Greek manuscripts in Diels. The identifications reproduce those in Touwaide 2016.

Finding Aid

City and Library names

Άγιον Όρος[2]: lxvii
Ιερά Μονή Διονυσίου: lxvii
Ιερά Μονή Δοχειαρίου: lxvii
Ιερά Μονή Εσφιγμένου: lxvii
Ιερά Μονή Ιβήρων: lxvii
Ιερά Μονή Παντελεήμονος: lxvii
Ιερά Μονή Ξηροποτάμου: lxviii
Antwerpen, Erfgoedbibliotheek Hendrik Conscience: lxviii
Αθήνα: lxviii
Βιβλιοθήκη της Βουλής των Ελλήνων: lxviii
Εθνική Βιβλιοθήκη της Ελλάδος ΕΒΕ: lxviii
Μετόχιον Παναγίου Τάφου-ΜΠΤ: lxviii

Berlin, Staatsbibliothek zu Berlin – Preussischer Kulturbesitz SBB-PKB: lxviii
Ms. graec. fol.: lxviii
Ms. graec. qu.: lxviii
Ms. Phill.: lxviii
Bern, Burgerbibliothek Bern/Bibliothèque de la Bourgeoisie de Berne: lxix
Bologna, Biblioteca Universitaria: lxix
Bruxelles, Bibliothèque royale de Belgique: lxix

Cambridge: lxix
Gonville and Caius College: lxix
University Library: lxix
Città del Vaticano, Biblioteca Apostolica Vaticana: lxix
Barberiniani: lxix
Ottoboniani: lxix
Palatini: lxx
Reginenses: lxx
Rossiani: lxx
Urbinates: lxx
Vaticani: lxx

Erlangen, Universitätsbibliothek Erlangen-Nürnberg: lxxi

Firenze: lxxi
Biblioteca Marucelliana: lxxi
Biblioteca Medicea Laurenziana: lxxi
Antinori: lxxi
Conventi soppressi: lxxi
plutei: lxxi
Biblioteca nazionale Magliabechiana: lxxii
Biblioteca Riccardiana: lxxii

Göttingen, Niedersächsische Staats- und Universitätsbibliothek: lxxii
Hist. nat.: lxxii
Philol.: lxxii

Heidelberg, Universitätsbibliothek: lxxiii

Ιερουσαλήμ, Πατριαρχείο, Πατριαρχική Βιβλιοθήκη: lxxiii
Ιερά Μονή Αγίου Σάββα: lxxiii
Πανάγιος Τάφος: lxxiii
Istanbul, Οικουμενικό Πατριαρχείο Κωνσταντινουπόλεως, Πατριαρχική Βιβλιοθήκη, Ιερά Μονή Παναγίας Καμαριωτίσσης: lxxiii

Jena, Thüringer Universitäts- und Landesbibliothek: lxxiii

Καλλονή Λέσβου, Βιβλιοθήκη τῆς τοῦ Λειμῶνος Μονῆς: lxxiii
Karlsruhe, Badische Landesbibliothek Karlsruhe: lxxiii
København, Det Kongelige Bibliotek, GkS: lxxiii

Leiden, Universiteitsbibliotheek: lxxiv
Bibliothecae Publicae Graecae (BPG): lxxiv
Scaligeriani (SCA): lxxiv
Vossiani graeci: lxxiv
folio (VGF): lxxiv
octavo (VGO): lxxiv
quarto (VGQ): lxxiv
Vossiani miscellanei (VMI): lxxiv

[2] Actually Μοναστική Πολιτεία Αγίου Όρους.

Vulcaniani (VUL): lxxiv
Leipzig, Universitätsbibliothek «Bibliotheca Albertina», Cod. graec.: lxxiv

London, British Library: lxxiv
Additional: lxxiv
Arundeliani: lxxiv
Harleiani: lxxiv
Royal: lxxv
Stowe: lxxv
London, Wellcome Library: lxxv

Madrid, Biblioteca nacional: lxxv
Milano: lxxv
Archivio Storico Civico e Biblioteca Trivulziana: lxxv
Biblioteca Ambrosiana: lxxv
Modena, Biblioteca Estense Universitaria: lxxvi
Москва (Moskva): lxxvi
Государственный Исторический Музей (ГИМ), Синодальная библиотека Московского Патриархата (Gosudarstvennyi Istoricheskii Muzei (GIM), Sinodal'naia Biblioteka Moskovskogo Patriarchata [State Historical Museum [GIM], Synodal Library of Moscow Patriarchate]), Синод. (Sinod.): lxxvi
München, Bayerische Staatsbibliothek, *graeci*: lxxvi

Napoli: lxxvii
Biblioteca Nazionale Vittorio Emanuele III: lxxvii
Biblioteca statale oratoriana del Monumento nazionale dei Girolamini: lxxvii
New Haven, Yale University
Harvey Cushing/John Hay Whitney Medical Library: lxxvii

Oxford: lxxvii
Bodleian Library: lxxvii
Ashmole: lxxvii
Auctarium: lxxvii
Barocci: lxxvii
Canon. Gr.: lxxvii
Clarkian.: lxxvii
Holkham: lxxviii
Ger. Langbainii Advers.: lxxviii
Marshall: lxxviii
D'Orville: lxxviii
Roe: lxxviii
Christ Church Library: lxxviii

Palermo, Biblioteca centrale della Regione siciliana «Alberto Bombace»: lxxviii
Paris : lxxviii
Bibliothèque Interuniversitaire de Santé-BIU Santé: lxxviii
Bibliothèque Mazarine: lxxviii
Bibliothèque nationale de France: lxxviii
Coisliniani: lxxviii
graeci: lxxviii
Supplément grec: lxxxi
Pistoia, Biblioteca Capitolare Fabroniana: lxxxi

Roma: lxxxi
Biblioteca Angelica: lxxxi
Biblioteca Corsiniana, Accademia dei Lincei: lxxxi
Biblioteca Vallicelliana: lxxxi

San Lorenzo de El Escorial, Monastery Library: lxxxii
Sens, Bibliothèque municipale: lxxxii

Torino, Biblioteca Nazionale Universitaria: lxxxii
Tübingen, Univivesitätsbibliothek: lxxxii

Uppsala, Uppsala Universitet: lxxxii

Venezia, Biblioteca Nazionale Marciana: lxxxiii
graeci: lxxxiii
appendix graeca: lxxxiii

Wien, Österreichische Nationalbibliothek: lxxxiii
historici: lxxxiii
latini: lxxxiii
medici: lxxxiii
philosophici et philologi graeci: lxxxiv
Supplementum graecum: lxxxiv
theologici: lxxxiv
Wolfenbüttel, Herzog August Bibliothek Wolfenbüttel: lxxxiv

Zürich, Zentralbibliothek Zürich-Kantons-, Stadt- und Universitätsbibliothek: lxxxiv

Index of Manuscripts

Άγιον Όρος, Ιερά Μονή Διονυσίου
See Athos, Βιβλ. Μον. Διονυσίου
59: 6 (3701.167)
465: 6 (3758.224)

Άγιον Όρος, Ιερά Μονή Δοχειαρίου
243 (2917): 7 (Athos, Βιβλ. Μον. Δοχειαρίου, 2917.243)

Άγιον Όρος, Ιερά Μονή Εσφιγμένου
See Athos, Βιβλ. Μον. Ἐσφιγμένου
310 (2323): 7 (2323.310)
317 (2330): 7 (2330.317)

Άγιον Όρος, Ιερά Μονή Ιβήρων
See Athos, Βιβλ. Μον. Ἰβήρων
92 (792): 7 (4212.92)
151 (4271): 7 (4271.151)
174 (4294): 8 (4294.174)
182 (4302): 8 (4302.182)
184 (4304): 8 (4304.184)
189 (4309): 8 (4309.189)
190 (4310): 8 (4310.190)
210 (4330): 8 (4330.310)
218 (4338): 8 (4338.218)
220 (4340): 8 (4340.220)
343 (4463): 9 (4463.343)
381 (4501): 9 (4501.381)
535 (4655): 9 (4655.535)
551 (4671): 9 (4671.551)
914 (5034): 9 (5034.914)

Άγιον Όρος, Ιερά Μονή Παντελεήμονος
See Athos, Βιβλ. Μον. Παντελεήμονος
262 (5769): 9 (5769.262)
289 (5796): 9 (5796.289)
835 (6342): 10 (6342.835)

Άγιον Όρος, Ιερά Μονή Ξηροποτάμου
    99 (2432): 10 (Athos, Βιβλ. Μον. Ξηροποτάμου, 2432.99)

Antwerpen, Erfgoedbibliotheek Hendrik Conscience
    B. 426: 5 (Antwerpen, Stadtbibliothek 426)

Αθήνα, Βιβλιοθήκη της Βουλής των Ελλήνων
See Athen, Βιβλ. τῆς Βουλῆς
    39: 5
    68: 5

Αθήνα, Εθνική Βιβλιοθήκη της Ελλάδος EBE
See Athen, Nationabibl.
    1477: 6
    1486: 6
    1488: 6
    1498: 6
    1500: 6
    1504: 6

Αθήνα, Εθνική Βιβλιοθήκη της Ελλάδος EBE
    Μετόχιον Παναγίου Τάφου – ΜΠΤ
    189: 27

Berlin, Staatsbibliothek zu Berlin – Preussischer Kulturbesitz SBB-PKB
See Berlin, Königl. Bibl.
    Ms. graec. fol.
        39: 10 (fol. 39 [275])
    Ms. graec. quart.
        5: 10 (qu. 5 [304])
    Ms. Phill.
        1462: 10
        1487: 11
        1524: 11 (1524 [ol. Meerm. 214])
        1525: 11 (1525 [ol. Meerm. 215])
        1527: 11 (1527 [ol. Meerm. 217])
        1529: 11 (1529 [ol. Meerm. 220])
        1532: 11 (1532 [ol. Meermann. 225])
        1533: 11
        1537: 12 (1537 [ol. Meerman. 233])
        1538: 12 (1538 [ol. Meerm. 233])

1566: 12 (1566 [ol. Meerm. 269])
1583: 12

Bern, Burgerbibliothek Bern/Bibliothèque de la Bourgeoisie de Berne
See Bern, Stadtbibliothek
579: 12

Bologna, Biblioteca Universitaria
3232: 12
3563: 12
3632: 12
3633: 13
3636: 13

Bruxelles, Bibliothèque royale de Belgique
See Brüssel, Königl. Bibl.
1871–77: 12
11345–48: 12

Cambridge, Gonville and Caius College
See Cambridge, Caius Coll.
50/27: 14 (50)
76/43: 14 (76), 15 ([949])
355/582: 15 (355)

Cambridge, University Library
See Cambridge, Cantabrig., Bibl. Univ.
Ii. 2. 5: 15 ([2239])
Kk. 5. 7: 15 (2049 [Kk V 7])
Ll. 4. 12: 15 (L. l IV 12)
Ll. 5. 4: 15 (L. L. 5, 4)

Città del Vaticano, Biblioteca Apostolica Vaticana
See Rom, Bibl. Vaticana
Barberiniani
See Rom, Bibl. Barberin.
5: 91 (I 5)
11: 91 (I 11 [= 136]), 92 (136 [= I 11])
127: 91 (I 127), 92 (276)
344: 92 (III 63 [= 245])
Ottoboniani
150: 93

157 A: 93
157 B: 93
192: 93
Palatini
126: 93
128: 93
129: 93
132: 94
143: 94
155: 94
157: 94
173: 94
192: 94
199: 95
278: 95
279: 95
297: 96
363: 96
385: 96
398: 96
400: 96
428: 96
Reginenses
See Reg. Suec.
173: 94 (Palat. 173), 96 (Reg. Suec. 173)
175: 97 (Reg.Suec. 175)
181: 97 (Reg. Suec. 181)
182: 97
Rossiani
982: 114 (Wien, Bibl.Colleg. S. J. Rossianus, XI.167)
Urbinates
64: 97
65: 98
67: 98
68: 98
Vaticani
276: 100
277: 101
278: 100 ([Vatic. 216]), 102 (Vatic. 278)
279: 103 (Vatic. 279)
280: 104

283: 104
285: 104
293: 104
294: 104
690: 104
876: 104
1062: 104
1063: 104
1065: 105
1066: 105
1095: 105
1133: 105 (1133 [Kl.])
1276: 105
1309: 105
1354: 105
1467: 105
1759: 105
1858: 105
1879: 106
2154: 106
2238: 106
2254: 106
2304: 106 (2304 [olim 2217])

Erlangen, Universitätsbibliothek Erlangen-Nürnberg
See Erlangen, Universitätsbibliothek
Ms A. 3: 16 (Erlangens. 90)

Firenze, Biblioteca Marucelliana
See Florenz, Bibl. Marucell.
A 109: 18

Firenze, Biblioteca Medicea Laurentiana
See Florenz, Bibl. Mediceo Laurentiana
Antinori
101: 23 (Laurent. App. 2)
Conventi soppressi
153: 19
plutei (Laurent. plut.)
plut. 59, 14: 19
plut. 71, 1: 19

plut. 74, 1: 19 ([plut. 25, ?]), 19 (plut., 74, 1)
plut. 74, 3: 21
plut. 74, 7: 21
plut. 74, 8: 21
plut. 74, 10: 21
plut. 74, 11: 21
plut. 74, 12: 22 ([plut. 74, 12])
plut. 74, 13: 22
plut. 74, 21: 22
plut. 74, 25: 22
plut. 74, 31: 22
plut. 75, 3: 22
plut. 75, 4: 19 ([plut. 25 ?])
plut. 75, 5: 22
plut. 75, 10: 23 (plut. 75, 10) ([plut. 75, 10])
plut. 75, 19: 23
plut. 75, 21: 23
plut. 75, 22: 23

Firenze, Biblioteca nazionale Magliabechiana
See Florenz, bibl. naz. [Magliabecchiana], and Magliabech.
Magliabechiani
1: 24 (bibl. naz. [Magliabecchiana] II.III.428), (Bibl. Magliabech. 1)

Firenze, Biblioteca Riccardiana
See Florenz, Bibl. Riccardiana, Riccard.
17: 24 (17 [K I 24])
41: 24 (41 [K II 2])
44: 24 b(44 [K II 5])

Göttingen, Niedersachsische Staats- und Universitätsbibliothek
See Göttingen, Univ.-Bibl.
Hist. nat.
4° Cod. Ms. hist. nat. 3: 25 (Hist. nat. 3)
4° Cod. Ms. hist. nat. 4: 25 (Hist. nat. 4)
4° Cod. Ms. hist. nat. 5: 25 (Hist. nat. 5)
Philol.
8° Cod. Ms. philol. 2: 25 (Philol. 2)
8° Cod. Ms. philol. 21: 25 (Philol. 21)

Heidelberg, Universitätsbibliothek
See Heidelberg, Bibl. Univ.
Cod. Pal. graec.
132: 25 (Bibl. Univ. 132)
155: 26 (Bibl. Univ. 155)
398: 26 (bibl. Univ. 398)

Ιερουσαλήμ, Πατριαρχείο, Πατριαρχική Βιβλιοθήκη
Ιερά Μονή Αγίου Σάββα
See Jerusalem, Bibl. Mar-Saba
432: 27
481: 27
498: 28
Πανάγιος Τάφος
See Jerusalem, Bibl. patriarch.
102: 28
148: 28
463: 28

Istanbul, Οικουμενικό Πατριαρχείο Κωνσταντινουπόλεως, Πατριαρχική Βιβλιοθήκη
Ιερά Μονή Παναγίας Καμαριωτίσσης
82: 16 (Chalke, Βιβλ. μον. Θεοτόκου 82)

Jena, Thüringer Universitäts- und Landesbibliothek
See Jena, Universitätsbibliothek
Ms. G.B. f. 31: 44 ([Moskau, Synodialbibl., ?])

Καλλονή Λέσβου, Βιβλιοθήκη τῆς τοῦ Λειμῶνος Μονῆς
See Lesbos, Βιβλ. τῆς τοῦ Λειμῶνος Μονῆς
175: 31

Karlsruhe, Badische Landesbibliothek Karlsruhe
See Karlsruhe, Großherzogl. Hof. u. Landesbibliothek
K 449: 28 (449)

København, Det Kongelige Bibliotek
See Kopenhagen, Königl. Bibliothek, and Bibl. Univ.
GkS
224, 2°: 29 (Königl. Bibliothek, Hauniens. ant. fund. reg. 224)

Leiden, Universiteitsbibliotheek
See Leyden, Universitäts-Bibliothek
Bibliothecae Publicae Graecae (BPG)
BPG 67 O: 31 (B. P. 670)
Scaligeriani (SCA)
SCA 71: 31
Vossiani graeci folio (VGF)
VGF 10: 32 (Voss. fol. 10)
Vossiani graeci octavo (VGO)
VGO 7: 32 (Voss. 8° 7)
Vossiani graeci quarto (VGQ)
VGQ 38: 32 (Voss. 4° 38)
VGQ 50: 32 (Voss. 4° 50)
Vossiani miscellanei (VMI)
VMI 1: 33 (Voss. Miscell. 1 pars 13)
Vulcaniani (VUL)
VUL 56: 33 (Vulc. 56)
VUL 108: 33 (Vulc. 108 pars 15)

Leipzig, Universitätsbibliothek «Bibliotheca Albertina»
See Leipzig, Universitätsbibliothek
Cod. graec.
56: 30
59: 30
61: 31
64: 31

London, British Library
See London, British Museum
Additional
See Addit. or Adit. (Brit. Mus.)
6898: 33
28,830: 33
34,060: 34
Arundeliani
538: 34
Harleiani
5611: 34
5626: 34
5635: 34
6295: 34

6301: 35
Royal
16.C.xvi: 35
Stowe
1073: 135

London, Wellcome Library
MS. MSL
See London, Medical Society
14: 35 (AA a 1 = Xa 32)
52 A&B: 35 (HH i 21. 22 = We 28. 29)
60: 35 (HHi 17 = We 30)

Madrid, Biblioteca nacional
See Madrid, Nationalbibliothek
4557: 36 (4557 [N 119])
4634: 36 (4634 [olim N 112])

Milano, Archivio Storico Civico e Biblioteca Trivulziana
685: 41(Mailand, Bibl. Trivulziana 685)

Milano, Biblioteca Ambrosiana
See Mailand, Bibl. Ambrosiana
A 45 sup.: 36
A 95 sup.: 36
A 110 sup.: 36
A 156 sup.: 36
B 72 sup.: 37
B 108 sup.: 37
B 113 sup.: 37
B 126 sup.: 37
C 4 sup.: 37
C 85 sup.: 38
C 119 sup.: 38 (C 118 Sup.), (C 119 Sup.)
F 23 sup.: 38
L 30 sup.: 39
L 110 sup.: 39
L 119 sup.: 38 (C 118 Sup.), (C 119 Sup.)
P 90 sup.: 39
Q 3 sup.: 40
Q 13 sup.: 40

S 19 sup.: 40
T 19 sup.: 40
A 27 inf.: 40
H 2 inf.: 40
S.Q.E.VIII.13: 40 (S.Q.E.VIII 13)
S.Q.T.VIII.9: 40 (S.Q.T.VIII 9)

Modena, Biblioteca Estense Universitaria
See Modena, Bibl. Estense
α.G.3.11: 42 (211 [III G 7])
α.G.3.12: 42 (213), (213 [III G 9])
α.J.6.28: 43(240 [III F 17])
α.N.8.8: 42 (191)
α.O.4.6: 42 (218 [II H 3])
α.O.4.8: 42 (220 [II H 5])
α.O.4.14: 42 (227 [II H 12])
α.P.5.17: 41 (115 [II D 16])
α.Q.5.16: 41 (85 [III C 6])
α.T.1.12: 43 (233 [III H 5])
α.U.9.3: 41 (54 [III B 2])
α.U.9.4: 41 (61 [III B 9])
α.W.3.12: 43 (237 [III G 18])

Москва (Moskva), Государственный Исторический Музей (ГИМ), Синодальная Библиотека Московского Патриархата (Gosudarstvennyi Istoricheskii Muzei (GIM), Sinodal'naja Biblioteka Moskovskogo Patriarchata [State Historical Museum [GIM], Synodal Library of Moscow Patriarchate])
Синод. (Sinod.)
See Moskau, Synodialbibl.
282: 44 (465)
283: 44 (466)
426: 44 (439)

München, Bayerische Staatsbibliothek
See München, Hof- und Staatsbibliothek
graeci
71: 45
72: 46
227: 46
231: 47
276: 47

287: 47
469: 47
494: 47
525: 47

Napoli, Biblioteca Nazionale Vittorio Emanuele III
See Neapel, Biblioteca Borbonica, and Neapel, Bibl. di S. Giovanni di Carbonara
II C 32: 48 (91 [II C 33]), 49 (Bibl. di S. Giovanni di Carbonara 15).
II F 30: 48 (187 [II F 30])
III AA 14bis: 49 (Bibl. di S. Giovanni di Carbonara 27)
III C 2: 48 (III C 2 [260])
III D 15: 147 (III D 15), 148 (229 [III D 15])

Napoli, Biblioteca statale oratoriana del Monumento nazionale dei Girolamini
Pil. XXII. n°. I: 48 (Neapel, Bibl. dei Gerolamini XXII.1), 49 (Neapel, Bibl. Oratoriana 152)

New Haven, Yale University, Harvey Cushing/John Hay Whitney Medical Library
Manuscript 50 vault: 121 (Zaragoza, Bibl. d. Cat. d. Pil. 1115 [olim 1427])

Oxford, Bodleian Library
See Oxford, Bibl. Bodleiana
Ashmole 1284: 13 ([Cambridge, Ashmol., 7751])
Auctarium
MS. Auct. F. inf. 2. 1: 53 (Miscell. 130)
MS. Auct. T. 2. 10: 50 (Auct. T II 10), 53 (Miscell. 210)
Barocci
See Baroccian.
10: 50
51: 50
76: 50
88: 50
131: 50
150: 50
204: 51
224: 52
Canon. Gr.
See Canonician.
1: 52
Clarkian.
MS. E.D. Clarke 16: 52 (16 [18378])

Holkham
See Holkham, Bibl. des Gr. Leicester
Gr. 92: 26 (Holkham 282), 54 ([Padua, Bibl. Canonicor. Lateranens]), (Padua, Bibl. S. Joannis in Viridario, ad dextr. plut. XVII)
Gr. 106: 27 (Holkham 293)
Ger. Langbainii Advers.
MS. Langbaine 2: 52
Marshall
MS. Marshall 72: 49 (Auct. F. Inf. II 3), 50 (Auct. T II 3), 53 (Miscell. 132)
D'Orville
See d'Orvillian.
MS. D'Orville 3: 5 ([Amsterdam, Universitäts-Bibliothek ?]), 53 (d'Orvillian. X 1. 1. 3)
MS. D'Orville 131: 53 (d'Orvillian. X 1. 4. 29)
Roe
14: 53 (Roe 14 [260]), 54 (Roe 14 [Bodl. 260]), (Roe XIV [260])

Oxford, Christ Church Library
See Oxford, Bibl. Aedis Christi
34: 49

Palermo, Biblioteca centrale della Regione siciliana «Alberto Bombace»
See Palermo, Biblioteca nazionale
XIII C 3: 55

Paris, Bibliothèque Interuniversitaire de Santé – BIU Santé
MS 44: 55 (Paris, Bibl. Facult. Med. 14), , 56 (Paris, Facult. Médic. 14), (Paris, Faculté de Méd.)

Paris, Bibliothèque Mazarine
4454: 55 (Paris, Bibl. de Paris 4)

Paris, Bibliothèque nationale de France
See Paris, Bibl. Nationale
Coisliniani (Coislin.)
163: 55 ([Paris, B. R. 120 ap. Montf. II 902]), 56
321: 56 (321), ([321 (?)])
335: 56 (Coislin. 335), 57 ([Coislin. 335])
graeci (Parisin.)
36: 57 (36), 88 ([3170])
396: 57

985: 57
1297: 57
1327: 57
1630: 58
1760: 58
1849: 58
1868: 58
1883: 59
1884: 58 ([1667 (?)]), ([1848 ?]), 59 (1884), ([1884]), ([1884 (?)]), ([1885]), ([1885 (?)])
1995: 60
2047: 60
2091: 60
2140: 57 ([1444 (?)]), 60 (2140), 61 ([2140]), 70 ([2146 (?)]
2141: 57 ([1444 (?)]), 61 (2141), 63 ([2141])
2142: 57 ([1444 (?)]), 63 (2142), 64 ([2142]), 75 ([2242 (?)])
2143: 57 ([1444 (?)]), 64 (2143), 66 ([2143]), ([2143 (?)]), 71 ([2148])
2144: 57 ([1444 (?)]), 66 (2144), 67 ([2144]), 72 ([2154])
2145: 57 ([1444 (?)]), 68 (2145), 69 ([2145]), 72 ([2154]), 85 (2545 [? = 2545 ? cf. Kühn l.1]), ([2545 (?) = 2145 ?]), (2545 [? = 2145 ?])
2146: 57 ([1444 (?)]), 69 (2146), 70 ([2146]), ([2146 (?)]), 86 ([2546 (? = 2146 ?)])
2147: 70 (2147), ([2147]), 71 ([2147 (?)])
2149: 71 (2149), 72 (2149 [?])
2149 (?): 71 (2149), 72 (2149 [?])
2150: 72
2151: 72
2155: 72
2161: 72
2165: 72
2166: 72
2168: 73
2174: 73
2177: 73
2178: 73
2219: 73
2222: 73
2223: 74
2224: 74
2228: 74 (2228), 87 ([2228 (? = 2228)])
2229: 74 (2229), ([2229 (?)])

2232: 75 ([2232]), 83 (2332)
2240: 75 (2240), 87 ([2699 (?)])
2247: 75 (2247), ([2247])
2248: 75 (2248), 76 ([2248])
2253: 76 (2253), ([2253]), 114 ([Venedig, Bibl. S. Anton.])
2254: 76 (2254), 80 ([2257 (?)])
2255: 57 ([1444 (?)], 77 ([2254]), ([2254 (?)]), 78 (2255), 79 ([2255]), ([2255 (?)])
2256: 76 ([2250]), 80 (2256), 81 ([2266 (?)])
2257: 80 (2257), 87 ([3140 (?)])
2258: 76 ([2250]), 80 (2258)
2259: 76 ([2250]), 80 (2259)
2260: 80 (2260)
2266: 80 (2266), 81 ([2266 (?)])
2269: 81 (2269), ([2269])
2276: 81
2278: 81
2287: 82
2294: 82
2295: 82
2296: 82
2301: 82 (2301), ([2301 (?)])
2304: 82 (2304)
2308: 82
2315: 82
2316: 83
2317: 83
2320: 83
2330: 60 ([2030]), 83 (2330)
2332: 75 ([2232]), 83 (2332), ([2332])
2419: 84
2510: 85
2596: 86
2614: 86
2615: 86
2651: 86
2652: 86
2671: 86 (2671), 87 ([2671 (?)])
2755: 87
2847: 87
2894: 87

3047: 87
3050: 87
3052: 87
Supplément grec
2: 88
64: 88
165: 88
205: 88
270: 88
352: 88
446: 88
447: 89 (447), 118 (Wien, Hofbibl. Vindob. med. 34)
496: 89
608: 89
637: 89 (637), (675)
675 : 89 (637), (675)
682: 89
684: 89
688: 90
1194: 90
1254: 90 (728 [Minas IZ]), (754 [Minas]), (1254)

Pistoia, Biblioteca Capitolare Fabroniana
See Pistoja, Biblioteca Fabroniana
Ms 308: 90 (141 [308])

Roma, Biblioteca Angelica
See Rom, Bibl. Angelica
Ang. gr. 4: 91 (4 [C.4.16])
Ang. gr. 80: 91 (80 [C.1.11])

Roma, Biblioteca Corsiniana, Accademia dei Lincei
See Rom, Bibl. Corsiniana (= Acc. d. Lincei)
Corsin. 36.E.26: 92 (1410 [36. E. 26])

Roma, Biblioteca Vallicelliana
See Rom, Bibl. Vallicellana
F 9: 92 (78 [F 9])
F 83: 93 (1106 [F 83])

San Lorenzo de El Escorial
See Escurial
Σ. II. 5: 16
Σ. II. 10: 16
Σ. II. 11: 16
T. II. 12: 17
T. II. 14: 17
Υ. III. 10: 17
Υ. III. 17: 17 (Υ III 17), (Υ. III. 17)
y. I. 8: 17
y. I. 9: 17
y. III. 16: 17
Φ. I. 10: 18
Φ. III. 7: 18
Φ. III. 11: 18
Φ. III. 12: 18
Ψ. III. 17: 18
Sens, Sens, Bibliothèque municipale, 187: 106

Torino, Biblioteca Nazionale Universitaria
See Turin, Bibl. Nationale (Universitaria)
B. V. 16: 107 (177 b II 31)
B. V. 33: 107 (179 b II 33), (B V 33 [179 b II 33])
C. VI. 3: 107 (287 c I 42), 108 (C VI 3 [287 c I 42])
C. VI. 10: 107 (156 b II 10)
C. VI. 21: 108 (C VI 21 [b VI 18])

Tübingen, Universitätsbibliothek
See Tübingen, Univ.-Bibl.
Mb 23: 106 (23)
Mb 37: 107 (37)

Uppsala, Uppsala Universitet
See Upsala, Upsal. bibl. acad.
Gr
8: 108 (8 (e don. Jo. Gabr. Sparfwenf. 49)
34: 108 (34)

Venezia, Biblioteca Nazionale Marciana
See Venedig, Bibl. National Marciana
graeci
269 (coll. 533): 108 ([Marcian.]), 109 ([Marcian.]), ([Marcian. ?]), (269)
277 (coll. 630): 110 (277)
278 (coll. 873): 110 (278)
279 (coll. 705): 111 (279)
281 (coll. 581): 111 (281)
282 (coll. 648): 111 (282)
283 (coll. 631): 109 ([Marcian. ap. Montfaucon, I 472]), 111 (283)
285 (coll. 708): 111 (285)
296 (coll. 632): 112 (296)
609 (coll. 686): 112 (609)
appendix graeca
V.4 (coll. 544): 112 (V, 4)
V.5 (coll. 1053): 112 (V, 5)
V.9 (coll. 1017): 112 (V, 9)
V.10 (coll. 1444): 113 (V, 10)
V.13 (coll. 1221): 113 (V, 13)
V.14 (coll. 1408): 113 (V, 14), (V, 14 [ol. Nanian. 248])
V.15 (coll. 1299): 113 (V, 15)
V.16 (coll. 1318): 113 (V, 16)
V.19 (coll. 986): 114 (V, 19)

Wien, Österreichische Nationalbibliothek
See Wien, Hofbibliothek
* 69. B. 101: 115 (Vindobon. 69 B 101)
historici
130: 114 ([Venedig, Bibl. S. Anton.]), 115 (130)
latini
4772: 116 (lat. 4772 [tab. cod. III 382])
medici
4: 115 ([Wien, Hofbilbiothek, Vindob. Lamb. VI 85]), 116 (med. 4)
8: 116 (med. 8), ([med. 8])
13: 116 (med. 13)
14: 116 (med. 14)
15: 115 ([Vindob. Ap. Nessel P. III]),([Vindob. 179]), 117 ([med. 15])
16: 117 (med. 16), (med. 16 [ol. 35])
24: 117 (med. 24)
28: 117 (med. 28), (med. [28 (?)])
31: 118 (med. 31)

32: 118 (med. 32)
34: 118 (med. 34)
38 [c]: 118 (med. 18 [c])
40: 118 (med. 40)
41: 118 (med. 41), 119 (med. [41])
43: 119 (med. 43)
44: 119 (med. 44)
47: 119 (med. 47)
48: 119 (med. 48)
49: 119 (med. 49)
52: 119 (med. 52)
53: 120 (53), ([53])
philosophici et philologi graeci
74: 120 (phil. 74)
82: 120 (phil. 82)
178: 120 (phil. 178)
179: 120 (phil. 179), 121 (philos. et philol. 179)
192: 121 (phil. 192)
219: 121 (phil. 219)
Supplementum graecum
179: 115 (Wien, Gollob Privatbesitz, Vindob.)
theologici
293: 121

Wolfenbüttel, Herzog August Bibliothek Wolfenbüttel
See Wolfenbüttel, Bibl. Guelf. August.
Augustei
18.1 Aug. 4°: 121 ([August. 18, 1]), (Guelferb. 3132 [18.1 Aug. 4°])

Zürich, Zentralbibliothek Zürich – Kantons-, Stadt- und Universitätsbibliothek
See Zürich, Stadtbibliothek
Ms. C 136: 122 (C 136)

Catalogue of Manuscripts

Notes for consultation

The catalogue that follows collects and exactly reproduces all the data presented for each Hippocratic manuscript listed in the three issues of Diels, also including the commentaries and other relevant material[1]. Each manuscript received an entry in which data are divided in two major parts: identification (followed by possible annotations) and contents[2].

Identifications of the manuscripts comprise a city and library name, a collection when appropriate, and a shelfmark. City names are mostly in German, whereas library names are either in German or in the original language (and in the Greek alphabet for several, but not all, of the libraries in Greece). The library names used by Diels do not always follow the actual form they had in Diels' time and, whatever their exactness, they are often in an abbreviated form. Collection names are either those of the libraries (often in an abbreviated form) or Latin adjectives formed on the name of the city. Shelfmarks are those used when Diels was compiled or sometimes, earlier ones, or even both. For some manuscripts, erroneous shelfmarks provided in the first two issues of Diels are corrected in the *Nachtrag* (Supplement). In some cases, Diels does not provide a shelfmark, but only a reference to a citation in an earlier catalogue or a more recent publication. For several items, all or some of these data (specifically the shelfmarks) appear between brackets in Diels (sometimes also with a question mark within the brackets) to indicate that they are reproduced from Ackermann (1791 and 1796) or Littré (1839–1861)[3]. The year or, in most cases, the century of copy of the manuscripts follows. For several manuscripts this chronological indication varies from one occurrence to another. All such divergent estimates are provided here in chronological order. In the catalogue contained in this volume, all these data form the first line of the entry devoted to each manuscript; they are printed in boldface for the

1 The commentaries are those by Apollonius Citiensis, Damascius, Galen, Ioannes Alexandrinus, Meletius, Palladius, Stephanus Atheniensis, and Theophilus. The lexicological lists compiled by Erotianus and Galen, and the *Vita* by Soranus are also included, in addition to some *iatrosophia* including fragments of Hippocratic texts. Unless these texts are the only ones contained in the manuscripts listed here, in all other cases they are listed in a separate section of the description of the contents of the manuscripts, below the list of the Hippocratic texts. In both cases, the name of the author is printed in boldface for the purposes of clarity.

2 Only manuscripts that have been preserved and precisely identified are listed here. Items lost (already in Diels' time or later), destroyed (including because of the two World Wars), missing, or mentioned in Diels, but not precisely identified as per the *Census*, have been omitted. They appear, however, in the catalogue of manuscripts in tome 5.

3 See p. 2 in the 1905 issue for an explanation of the brackets.

purposes of easy and direct consultation. Notes about the possible untraceability and the state of preservation of some manuscripts, as well as possible corrections of shelfmark and time of copy provided in the *Nachtrag* (Supplement) are reproduced in the next line, printed in italic.

When necessary, the identification of the manuscripts is followed (on the next line) by annotations providing the correspondence between Diels' and current identification of the manuscripts since several Diels identifiers do not correspond to their actual or current equivalent (from the city names in German to possible changes of shelfmarks). Correspondences (particularly of shelfmarks) that could not be established with a degree of certainty are introduced by a question mark. All correspondences reproduce those provided in the *Census of Greek Medical Manuscripts* (2016), which is referenced between parentheses after the current identification. To avoid repetition among the entries when several manuscripts appear in the same library or collection, Diels' and current names are provided only once, at the beginning of the section of the catalogue devoted to the library or the collection.

A special case is that of the manuscripts listed in Diels under different shelfmarks or with a shelfmark between brackets. Each distinct shelfmark in Diels has received an entry. However, all such entries include a reference to the manuscripts they refer to and, conversely, they are referred to in the entry of the manuscripts they are related to. These cross-references follow the identification of the manuscripts (Diel's and current). Shelfmarks (or other identifiers) referred to are printed in boldface to allow for easy cross-referencing.

The second and most substantial part of each entry details the contents of the manuscripts. All the texts included in Diels (and only those) are listed here, with the following four descriptors: the folios where they appear or their sequential number in the manuscripts (in both cases between parentheses), the author's name for the commentaries and other relevant material[4], the title of the work (in italic), and any possible notes of commentary between parentheses (*incipit*, lacunae, *desinit*, source, comparison with other texts, or any other philological or textual peculiarity as identified in Diels, sometimes with the name of Diels' collaborator who provided the information). References to other manuscripts (sometimes without precise shelfmark in Diels) have been made explicit (via shelfmark between brackets) to allow for cross-referencing. The asterisk that follows the title of some works in Diels to indicate a fragmentary text has been replaced by the explicit mention *Frgm*. References to the parts and pages of Diels' catalogue, and mentions of collations made or owned by Diels' collaborators have been omitted, as have also been some historical notes.

4 Hippocrates' name has been systematically omitted, except in the case of some *iatrosophia*.

Amsterdam

[Amsterdam, Universitäts-Bibliothek, Amstelodam. ?].
= Oxford, Bodleian Library, MS. D'Orville 3 (*Census*: 9, nr [0001]) (below p. 53).

Galenos, *Linguarum sive dictionum exoletarum Hippocratis explicatio.*

Antwerpen

Antwerpen, Stadtbibliothek, Antverp. 426; s. XVI.
Now Antwerp, Erfgoedbibliotheek Hendrik Conscience, B. 426 (*Census*: 10, nr [0002]).

(f. 92^{v}) *Aphorismi.*

Athen, Βιβλ. τῆς Βουλῆς
Now Αθήνα, Βιβλιοθήκη της Βουλής των Ελλήνων

Athen, Βιβλ. τῆς Βουλῆς, 39; s. XVIII.

(f. 1) *De morbis I.*
(f. 1 sqq.) *De morbis II–III.*
(f. 1 sqq.) *De morbis liber IV.*
(f. 98^{v}) *De affectionibus.*
(f. 118^{v}) *De internis affectionibus.*
(f. 161^{v}) *De virginum morbis.*
(f. 163) *De natura muliebri* (Expl. καὶ ἣν ταῦτα φάγῃ ἢ πίῃ, ὡς πρὸς [sic] εἴπομεν, ὥστε ἀνάγκῃ ...).

Athen, Βιβλ. τῆς Βουλῆς, 68; s. XVIII.

(f. 109) *Prognostica* (Προγν. μυστηριώδη).
(f. 220) *De morbis* (Exc. varia περὶ παθῶν ex Hipp., Gal., Paulo Nic., Paulo Aeg.).
(f. 299) *Aphorismi* (Expl. mut. sect. II τὰ πάντα εἶναι ἀσθενέστερα · περὶ δὲ ...).

Athen, Nationalbibl.
Αθήνα, Εθνική Βιβλιοθήκη της Ελλάδος ΕΒΕ

Athen, Nationalbibl., 1477; s. XV; XVI.

De fracturis.
Opera varia (προηγεῖται τὸ π. ἀγμῶν).

Athen, Nationalbibl., 1486; a. 1793.

Aphorismi (Ἑρμηνεῖαι εἰς τοὺς ἀφ. καταστρωθεῖσαι εἰς κοινὴν φράσιν παρὰ Μπαλάνου Βασιλοπούλου).

Athen, Nationalbibl., 1488; s. XIX.

De morbis popularibus I et III (Lib. I).

Athen, Nationalbibl., 1498; s. XVIII.

Aphorismi (*Wie in* [Athen.] nr. 1486) (above).

Athen, Nationalbibl., 1500.

Aphorismi (Μάρκου τοῦ Κυπρίου Μετάφρασις τῶν Ἱππ. ἀφ. μετά τινος ἐπιστασίας καὶ ἑρμηνείας ἐκ τῆς τοῦ Γαλ. διδασκαλίας συλλεγείσης).

Athen, Nationalbibl., 1504; s. XIX.

Prognostica (Προγν. μυστηριώδη).

Athos, Βιβλ. Μον. Διονυσίου
Now Ἅγιον Ὄρος, Ιερά Μονή Διονυσίου

Athos, Βιβλ. Μον. Διονυσίου, 3701. 167; s. XV.
Now 59 (*Census*: 16, nr [0028]).

Ad Ptolemaeum regem epistula de hominis fabrica.

Athos, Βιβλ. Μον. Διονυσίου, 3758. 224; s. XVI.
Now 465 (*Census*: 16, nr [0030]).

(p. 985) *Hippocratis ad Galenum discipulum liber de pulsibus et de temperamentis corporis humani.*

Athos, Βιβλ. Μον. Δοχειαρίου
Now Άγιον Όρος, Ιερά Μονή Δοχειαρίου

Athos, Βιβλ. Μον. Δοχειαρίου, 2917. 243; s. XVII.
Now Άγιον Όρος, Ιερά Μονή Δοχειαρίου 243 (2917) (*Census*: 17, nr [0037]).

(f. 163 A) *Hippocratis ad Galenum discipulum liber de pulsibus et de temperamentis corporis humani* (Περὶ εἰς πίον τόπον τοῦ κορμίου τοῦ ἀνθρώπου εὑρίσκεται καθένα στοιχίον ἀπο τα τεσσαρα. Ἱπποκράτους πρ. Γαλ. τοῦ αὐτοῦ μαθητήν).

Athos, Βιβλ. Μον. Ἐσφιγμένου
Now Άγιον Όρος, Ιερά Μονή Εσφιγμένου

Athos, Βιβλ. Μον. Ἐσφιγμένου, 2323. 310; s. XVIII.
= 310 (2323) (*Census*: 18, nr [0039]).

Aphorismi.

Athos, Βιβλ. Μον. Ἐσφιγμένου, 2330. 317; s. XVI.
= 317 (2330) (*Census*: 18, nr [0040]).

De natura hominis.

Athos, Βιβλ. Μον. Ἰβήρων
Now Άγιον Όρος, Ιερά Μονή Ιβήρων

Athos, Βιβλ. Μον. Ἰβήρων, 4212. 92; s. XVI.
= 92 (792) (*Census*: 10, nr [0042]).

(f. 367 A) *Ad Ptolemaeum regem epistula de hominis fabrica.*

Athos, Βιβλ. Μον. Ἰβήρων, 4271. 151; s. XV.
= 151 (4271).

(f. 17 a) *Lexicon specierum.*
(f. 85 B) *Remedia* (Inscr. Ἡ ἱερὰ Ἱπποκράτους. Inc. Κολοκυνθίδι ἐντεριώνην σκίλλης ὀπτῆς ἀγαρικοῦ.

Athos, Βιβλ. Μον. Ἰβήρων, 4294. 174; s. XVII.
= 174 (4294) (*Census*: 19, nr [0046]).

(f. 46b [463 ?]) **Hippokrates, Galenos,** *Jatrosophium* (Ἰατροσόφιον ἐκλελεγμ. ὑπὸ πολλ. ἰατρικῶν βιβλίων Γαλ. Ἱππ. καὶ ἄλλων πολλ. σοφῶν ἰατρῶν).

Athos, Βιβλ. Μον. Ἰβήρων, 4302. 182; s. XVI.
= 182 (4302) (*Census*: 19, nr [0050]).

(f. 8 B) *Iusiurandum.*
(p. 9 b) *Hippocratis ad Galenum discipulum liber de pulsibus et de temperamentis corporis humani* (Λέξεις Ὑπποκράτους ἀρχιατροῦ πρ. τὸν αὐτοῦ μαθ. Γαλ.).

Athos, Βιβλ. Μον. Ἰβήρων, 4304. 184; s. XIV/XV.
= 184 (4304) (*Census*: 19, nr [0051]).

Galenos: (f. 130 A) *In Hippocratis librum de acutorum victu commentarii IV.*

Athos, Βιβλ. Μον. Ἰβήρων, 4309. 189; s. XIII.
= 189 (4309) (*Census*: 19, nr [0052]).

Galenos: (f. 42 A) *In Hippocratis librum de acutorum victu commentarii IV.*

Athos, Βιβλ. Μον. Ἰβήρων, 4310. 190; s. XIII.
= 190 (4310) (*Census*: 20, nr [0053]).

(f. 115 a) *Excerpta varia.*

Athos, Βιβλ. Μον. Ἰβήρων, 4330. 310; s. XVI.
= 210 (4330) (*Census*: 20, nr [0055]).

(f. 44 B) *Hippocratis ad Ptolemaeum regem epistula.*

Athos, Βιβλ. Μον. Ἰβήρων, 4338. 218; s. XVI.
= 218 (4338) (*Census*: 20, nr [0058]).

(p. 310) *De aloe.*

Athos, Βιβλ. Μον. Ἰβήρων, 4340. 220; s. XVII.
= 220 (4340) (*Census*: 21, nr [0060]).

De urinis.

Athos, Βιβλ. Μον. Ἰβήρων, 4463. 343; s. XIX.
= 343 (4463) (*Census*: 21, nr [0063]).

Jatrosophium (Ἱππ. ἰατρικὸν συνταγμάτιον).
Prognostica.

Athos, Βιβλ. Μον. Ἰβήρων, 4501. 381; s. XV.
= 381 (4501) (*Census*: 21, nr [0066]).

(f. 341 A) *Ad Ptolemaeum regem epistula de hominis fabrica*.

Athos, Βιβλ. Μον. Ἰβήρων, 4655. 535; s. XVI.
= 535 (4655) (*Census*: 21, nr [0068]).

Galenos, Hippokrates, Meletius monachus, *Iatrosophia/Excerpta varia* (Ἰατροσόφη ἐκλελεγμένον ὑπὸ ... Γαλ. Ἱππ. καὶ Μελ. καὶ ἄλλων δοκίμων ἰατρῶν. Cap. 1. Ὅτι ὁ κόσμος ὑπὸ τεσσάρων στοιχείων).

Athos, Βιβλ. Μον. Ἰβήρων, 4671. 551; s. XVII.
= 551 (4671) (*Census*: 21, nr [0069]).

Aphorismi (Frgm. Ἀφορισμοὶ ἀπὸ τοῦ Β' τμήματος τοῦ Ἱππ.).

Athos, Βιβλ. Μον. Ἰβήρων, 5034. 914; s. XVII.
= 914 (5034) (*Census*: 22, nr [0077]).

Ad Ptolemaeum regem epistula de hominis fabrica (Expl. εἰς ἡμέρας τξε' καὶ τέταρτον).

Athos, Βιβλ. Μον. Παντελεήμονος
Now Άγιον Όρος, Ιερά Μονή Παντελεήμονος

Athos, Βιβλ. Μον. Παντελεήμονος, 5769. 262; s. XVIII.
= 262 (5769) (*Census*: 25, nr [0093]).

Meletius monachus, Hippokrates, Galenos, Paulus Aegineta: (f. 15 [15 A]) *Excerpta varia* (Ἰατροσόφιον ἐκλελεγμένον ὑπὸ πολλῶν ἰατρικῶν βιβλ. Γαλ. Ἱππ. Μελ. καὶ Παύλ. τοῦ Αἰγ. συγγραφὲν δὲ παρὰ Κοσμᾶ ἱερομονάχου τοῦ Μακεδόνος).

Athos, Βιβλ. Μον. Παντελεήμονος, 5796. 289; s. XVIII.
= 289 (5696) (*Census*: 25, nr [0094]).

(p. 830) *Aphorismi* (Ἀφορισμοὶ ἀπὸ τοῦ β' τμήματος τοῦ Ἱππ.).

Athos, Βιβλ. Μον. Παντελεήμονος, 6342. 835; s. XVII.
= 835 (6342) (*Census*: 26, nr [0095]).

Aphorismi.

Athos, Βιβλ. Μον. Ξηροποτάμου
Now Άγιον Όρος, Ιερά Μονή Ξηροποτάμου

Athos, Βιβλ. Μον. Ξηροποτάμου, 2432. 99; s. XVII.
= 99 (2432) (*Census*: 26, nr [0099]).

De splene et stomacho.
Testamentum (Διαθήκη τῶν τριῶν ἰατρῶν Γαλ. Ἱππ. καὶ Διοσκορ.).

Berlin, Königl. Bibl.
Now Staatsbibliothek zu Berlin – Preussischer Kulturbesitz SBB-PKB

Berlin, Königl. Bibl., qu. 5 (304); s. XV/XVI.
Now Kraków, Biblioteka Jagiellońska, quarto 5 (*Census*: 33, nr [0152], 103).

(f. 53v) *Testamentum* (Διαθήκη τῶν τριῶν ἰατρῶν Γαλ. Ἱππ. καὶ Μελετ. περὶ τῆς τοῦ ἀνθρώπου κατασκευῆς καὶ πῶς δεῖ διεξιέναι τὸν καιρόν).

Berlin, Königl. Bibl., fol. 39 (275); s. –, XVIII–XIX, XIX.
= Ms. graec. fol. 39 (Census: 28, nr [0115]).

Erotianus, *Vocum Hippocraticarum conlectio.*

Berlin, Königl. Bibl., Phillipps.
Now Berlin, Staatsbibliothek zu Berlin – Preussischer Kulturbesitz SBB-PKB, Ms. Phill.

Berlin, Königl. Bibl., Phillipps. 1462; s. XV/XVI.
= Ms. Phill. 1462 (*Census*: 29, nr [0118]).

(f. 407) *Ad Ptolemaeum regem epistula de hominis fabrica.*

Berlin, Königl. Bibl., Phillipps. 1487; s. XV/XVI.
= Ms. Phill. 1487 (*Census*: 29, nr [0119]).

(p. 339) *Hippocratis ad Galenum discipulum liber de pulsibus et de temperamentis corporis humani* (Expl. ἡ τροφὴ αὐτοῦ ξηρὰ καὶ γλυκέα).

Berlin, Königl. Bibl., Phillipps. 1524 (ol. Meerm. 214); s. XV, XVI.
= Ms. Phill. 1524 (*Census*: 29, nr [0120]).

Theophilus: (f. 1) *Commentarius in Hippocratis aphorismos* (Inc. κείμενον · ὁ βίος βραχύς. Expl. ὅθεν ἡ ἔκλυσις γίνεται. »Codex verbis ab editione discrepat nec totum commentarium continet«).

Berlin, Königl. Bibl., Phillipps. 1525 (ol. Meerm. 215); s. XVI.
= Ms. Phill. 1525 (*Census*: 29, nr [0121]).

Galenos, *Linguarum sive dictionum exoletarum Hippocratis explicatio* (Expl. mutil. ψαφερον ψαδυρὸν ψέφαρα).
Palladius: (f. 1) *Scholia in Hippocratis de popularibus morbis librum sextum, sectiones VIII.*

Berlin, Königl. Bibl., Phillipps. 1527 (ol. Meerm. 217); s. XVI.
= Ms. Phill. 1527 (*Census*: 29, nr [0123]).

(f. 61) *De alimentorum differentiis.*

Berlin, Königl. Bibl., Phillipps. 1529 (ol. Meerm. 220); s. XVI.
= Ms. Phill. 1529 (*Census*: 30, nr [0125]).

(f. 194) *De septimanis* (Inc. Ἑπτά εἰσιν ὥραι. Expl. κἂν ἀτύχῃ τὰ τοῦτέλους; cf. L. VIII 633).

Berlin, Königl. Bibl., Phillipps. 1532 (ol. Meerman. 225); s. XVI.
= Ms. Phill. 1532 (*Census*: 30, nr [0128]).

(f. 154) *Aphorismi* (Anon. comm. in Hipp. Aph.).

Berlin, Königl. Bibl., Phillipps. 1533; s. XVII.
= Ms. Phill. 1533 (*Census*: 30, nr [0129]).

Apollonius Citiensis:
(f. 90) *Commentarius in Hippocratis de articulis, libri III* (Liber I).
(f. 121) *Commentarius in Hippocratis de articulis, libri III* (Liber II).
(f. 135) *Commentarius in Hippocratis de articulis, libri III* (Liber III).

Berlin, Königl. Bibl., Phillipps. 1537 (ol. Meerman. 233); s. XV.
= Ms. Phill. 1537 (*Census*: 30, nr [0133]).

(f. 199[v]) *Aphorismi* (Frgm.).

Berlin, Königl. Bibl., Phillipps. 1538 (ol. Meerm. 233); s. XV ex.
= Ms. Phill. 1538 (*Census*: 30, nr [0134]).

Excerpta varia.

Berlin, Königl. Bibl., Phillipps. 1566 (ol. Meerm. 269); s. XVI.
= Ms. Phill. 1566 (*Census*: 31, nr [0141]).

(f. 1) *Hippocratis ad Ptolemaeum regem epistula.*

Berlin, Königl. Bibl., Phillipps. 1583; s. XV.
= Ms. Phill. 1583 (*Census*: 32, nr [0150]).

(f. 94[v]) *Ad Ptolemaeum regem epistula de hominis fabrica.*

Bern, Stadtbibliothek
Now Burgerbibliothek Bern/Bibliothèque de la Bourgeoisie de Berne

Bern, Stadtbibliothek, 579; s. XIV.

(f. 61) *Epistulae* (Epp. 4–6).
(f. 98–99) *De insomniis* (Frgm.).

Bologna, Bibl. Universitaria

Bologna, Bibl. Universitaria, Bonon. 3232; s. XV.

(f. 28[v]) *Aphorismi* (Expl. λιμὸς γὰρ ξηραίνει τὰ σώματα).

Bologna, Bibl. Universitaria, Bonon. 3563; s. XVI.

(f. 89[v]) *Epistulae* (1–5. [6–9 man. alt. add. in marg.]. 11–18. 20. 22).

Bologna, Bibl. Universitaria, Bonon. 3632; s. XV.

(f. 27[v]) *De anatomicis ferramentis* (Περὶ ἀνατομικῶν ἐργαλίον κατὰ υπ̅π̅κ ποσα ἡσή ἡστὴν ἰατρικήν ἐπιστίμην).

(f. 28) *De prisca medicina* (Frgm.).
(f. 28) *Iusiurandum* (Frgm. »Ἐκ τοῦ κατὰ τὸν Ἱππ. ὅρκου, καθόσον οἷόν τε Χριστιανῶι ὀμόσαι«).
(f. 28) *De arte* (Frgm.).
(f. 28) *Lex* (Frgm.).
(f. 36) *Prognosticon.*
(f. 46) *De genitura.*
(f. 46 [post]) *De anatome.*
(f. 46 [post]) *Ad Ptolemaeum regem epistula de hominis fabrica.*

Apollonius Citiensis: (f. 419–434) *Commentarius in Hippocratis de articulis, libri III* (Imagines).

Bologna, Bibl. Universitaria, Bonon. 3633; s. XV.

(f. 126) *Hippocratis vel Dioclis epistula ad Ptolemaeum Aegypti regem.*

Bologna, Bibl. Universitaria, Bonon. 3636; s. XIV–XV.

(f. 151^v) *Aphorismi* (»explicatio locutionis Ἀφορισμὸς **Philothei**«).
(f. 152) *Aphorismi* (»cum scholiis«).

Brüssel, Königl. Bibl.
Now Bruxelles, Bibliothèque royale de Belgique

Brüssel, Königl. Bibl., Bruxell. 1871–77; s. –.

(f. 68) *Epistulae.*

Brüssel, Königl. Bibl., Bruxell. 11345–48; s. XVI.

Erotianus: (f. 1) *Vocum Hippocraticarum conlectio.*
Galenos: (f. 25) *Linguarum sive dictionum exoletarum Hippocratis explicatio.*

Cambridge

[Cambridge, Ashmol., 7751; s. –].
= Oxford, Bodleian Library, MS. Ashmole 1284 (*Census*: 39–40, nr [0182]).

Prognosticon.

Cambridge, Caius Coll.
Now Cambridge, Gonville and Caius College

Cambridge, Caius Coll., 50; s. XV/XVI.
Now 50/27 (*Census*: 40, nr [0184]).

(f. 1) *Iusiurandum.*
(f. 1^v) *Lex.*
(f. 2) *Esse re vera artes.*
(f. 2) *De arte.*
(f. 2^v) *De substantia artis medicae. Definitio artis medicae.*
(f. 6^v) *De prisca medicina.*
(f. 15^v) *Praeceptiones.*
(f. 18) *De decenti ornatu.*
(f. 21) *De natura hominis.*
(f. 27 b) *De salubri diaeta.*
(f. 30^v) *De genitura.*
(f. 33^v) *De natura pueri.*
(f. 45^v) *De articulis.*
(f. 81^v) *De humoribus.*
(f. 86) *De alimento.*
(f. 88) *De ulceribus.*
(f. 94) *De morbo sacro.*
(f. 102) *De morbis I.*
(f. 102) *De morbis II et III.*
(f. 102) *De morbis liber IV.*
(f. 159) *De affectionibus.*
(f. 199^v) *De victus ratione I–III.*
(f. 172) *De internis affectionibus.*
(f. 230^v) *De insomniis.*
(f. 234^v) *De visu.*
(f. 236) *De diebus iudicatoriis.*
(f. 238^v) *Aphorismi* (Expl. τὰ δ' ἐναντία δυσχερῶς. τέλος τοῦ α').

Soranus: (f. 1) *Hippocratis genus et vita secundum Soranum.*

Cambridge, Caius Coll., 76; s. XV/XVI.
Now 76/43 (*Census*: 40, nr [0185]).
See also [949] below.

(f. 206) *De ulceribus.*

(f. 213 [?]) *De officina medici.*
(f. 220) *De natura pueri* (Inc. ἡ τροφὴ καὶ ἡ αὔξησις τῶν παιδίων = L. VII 514, 6).

Cambridge, Caius Coll., 355; s. XV/XVI.
Now 355/582 (*Census*: 40, nr [0187]).

(f. 92) *Aphorismi* (Inc. ἐν δὲ τοῖσι παροξυσμοῖς. Expl. μᾶλλον βλάψεις sect. 7).
(f. 117) *Prognosticon.*
(f. 120) *Aphorismi* (Inc. ἐν δὲ τοῖσι παροξυσμοῖς. Expl. μᾶλλον βλάψεις sect. 7).

[Cambridge, Caius Coll., 949; s. –].
= part of **76/43** above (*Census*: 42, nr [0191]).
Now 76/43.

De ulceribus.

Cambridge, Cantabrig. Bibl. Univ.
Now Cambridge, University Library

Cambridge, Cantabrig. Bibl. Univ., 2049 (Kk V 7); s. XV–XVI.
Now Cambridge University Library Kk. 5. 7 (*Census*: 44–45, nr [0197]).

Erotianus, *Vocum Hippocraticarum conlectio.*

[Cambridge, Cantabrig. Bibl. Univ., 2329; s. –].
Now Cambridge University Library Ii. 2. 5 (*Census*: 45, nr [0198]).

Prognosticon.

Cambridge, Cantabrig. Bibl. Univ., L l IV 12; s. XV.
Now Cambridge University Library Ll. 4. 12.

(f. 39 b) *Epistulae* (Ep. 17 Frgm. et 18).
(f. 39) *De insomniis.*
(f. 40) *De natura hominis* (Frgm.).
(f. 40^{v}) *De victus ratione I–III.*

Cambridge, Cantabrig. Bibl. Univ., L. L. 5, 4; s. – (»très moderne«).
Now Cambridge University Library Ll. 5. 4.

De officina medici.

Chalke

Chalke, Βιβλ. μον. Θεοτόκου, 82; s. –.
Now Istanbul, Οικουμενικό Πατριαρχείο Κωνσταντινουπόλεως, Πατριαρχική Βιβλιοθήκη, Ιερά Μονή Παναγίας Καμαριωτίσσης, 82 (*Census*: 50, nr [0211]).

(f. 188ᵛ) *Hippocratis ad Ptolemaeum regem epistula.*

Erlangen, Universitätsbibliothek
Now Universitätsbibliothek Erlangen-Nürnberg

Erlangen, Universitätsbibliothek, 90 (vel Erlangens. 90); s. XVI.
Now Ms A. 3 (*Census*: 61, nr [0235]).

Aphorismi (»Addita est inde ab *Aph.* XXIV. explicatio **Philothei.**« Inc. Τὰ διακαῆ καὶ ζέουσαν. Expl. τέλος τῶν λειπομένων Θεοφίλου φιλοσ. εἰς τοῦ Ἱππ. ἀφορισμούς).

Theophilus: (nr. 90) *Commentarius in Hippocratis aphorismos* (Inde ab aphor. XXIV).

Escurial
Now San Lorenzo de El Escorial,
Biblioteca del Real Monastero de San Lorenzo del Escorial

Escurial, Scorial. Σ. II. 5; s. XV.

(f. 28ᵛ) *Iusiurandum.*

Galenos: (f. 73 *und* 178–183) *In Hippocratis librum de acutorum victu commentarii IV.*

Escurial, Scorial. Σ. II. 10; s. X.

Stephanus Atheniensis: (f. 1) *In aphorismos Hippocratis commentarius* (Inc. ⟨Αἱ⟩ μεταβολαὶ τῶν ὡρέων. Expl. φύσει ἀνώμαλον εἶναι τὸ φθινόπωρον).

Escurial, Scorial. Σ. II. 11; s. XV.

Galenos: (f. 32) *In Hippocratis de humoribus librum commentarii III.*

Escurial, Scorial. Τ. II. 12; s. XVI.

(f. 190) *De urinis.*

Escurial, Scorial. Τ. II. 14; s. XVII.

(f. 235) *De insomniis* (Expl. ἐς τὴν ἔσω περιφορὴν ἐμπεπτωκέναι).

Escurial, Scorial. Υ. III. 10; s. XV.

(f. 26[v]) *Hippocratis ad Galenum discipulum liber de pulsibus et de temperamentis corporis humani* (Expl. *wie im* Berol. Phill. [1487]) (p. 11).

Escurial, Scorial. Υ III 17; s. XVI.
Same as **Y. III. 17** below (*Census*: 64 nr [0256]).

(f. 135) *Prognosticon* (c. comm. Gal.).

Escurial, Scorial. Υ. III. 17; s. XVI.
See also **Y III 17** above.

Galenos: (f. 127) *Hippocratis aphorismi et Galeni in eos commentarii VII.*
Galenos: (f. 135) *In Hippocratis prognosticum commentarii III.*

Escurial, Scorial. y. I. 8; s. XVI.

(f. 1) *Aphorismi.*
(f. 1) *Lex.*
(f. 1) *Qualem oporteat esse discipulum.*
(f. 2) *Iusiurandum.*

Theophilus: (f. 1) *Commentarius in Hippocratis aphorismos.*
Palladius: (f. 82) *Scholia in Hippocratis de popularibus morbis librum sextum, sectiones VIII.*

Escurial, Scorial. y. I. 9; s. XVI.

Erotianus: (f. 158) *Vocum Hippocraticarum conlectio.*

Escurial, Scorial. y. III. 16; s. XV.

(f. 1) *De septimanis* (Frgm. Inc. εἰσὶ δὲ ἡλικίαι ἑπτά, ὥς φησιν Ἱππ.; cf. L. VIII 636).

Escurial, Scorial. Φ. I. 10; s. XVI.

(f. 196ᵛ) *De elementis* (*Wie im* Neapolit. [Gerolamini XXII.I]) (below p. 48).

Escurial, Scorial. Φ. III. 7; s. XIV.

(f. 9) *Prognosticon* (c. comm. Gal.).
(f. 67) *Aphorismi* (cum comm. Gal.).

Galenos:
(f. 9) *In Hippocratis prognosticum commentarii III.*
(f. 67) *Hippocratis aphorismi et Galeni in eos commentarii VII.*

Escurial, Scorial. Φ. III. 11; s. XIV–XV, XIV. XV, XIV *und* **XV.**

(f. 43) *Qualem oporteat esse discipulum* (Inc. πρῶτον μὲν τῷ γένει ἐλεύθερον. Expl. εἰ μὴ μόνον ἡμῖν τοῖς ἰατροῖς).

Escurial, Scorial. Φ. III. 12; s. XV.

(f. 8) *De urinis.*
(f. 9) *Prognosticon* (Exc.).
(f. 443ᵛ) *Aphorismi.*
(f. 457) *Prognosticon.*
(f. 461) *De flatibus.*

Escurial, Scorial. Ψ. III. 17; s. XVI.

(f. 23) *Aphorismi* (cum comm. anon.).
(f. 127) *Aphorismi* (cum comm. **Galenos**).

Florenz, Bibliotheca Marucelliana
Firenze, Biblioteca Marucelliana

Florenz, Bibl. Marucell., A 109; s. –.
= Firenze, Biblioteca Marucelliana, A 109.

Lex.

Florenz, Bibl. Mediceo Laurentiana
Firenze, Biblioteca Medicea Laurenziana

Florenz, Bibl. Mediceo Laurentiana, Conventi soppressi 153; XVI.

(f. 74) *Epistulae* (Epp. 1–5. 11–18. 20. 22).

[Florenz, Bibl. Mediceo Laurentiana, Laurent. plut. 25, ?].
= **plut. 74, 1** below (*Census*: 69–70, nr [0290]).

Praesagiorum liber I.

[Florenz, Bibl. Mediceo Laurentiana, Laurent. plut. 25, ?].
= **plut. 75, 4** (*Census*: 69–70, nr [0291]).

Praesagiorum liber II.

Florenz, Bibl. Mediceo Laurentiana, Laurent. plut. 59, 14; s. XIII, XV.
Dieses Werk (= Philaretus, *De pulsibus*) *von einer Hand des XIII (!) Saec.*; f. 171^{v} (= Galenos, *De pulsibus ad Antonium*) *andere Hand*; *sonst* s. XV.

(f. 100^{v}) *Aphorismi* (Frgm.).
(f. 227 b) *De natura pueri* (Frgm. c. comm. **Joannis [Damasceni ?]**. Ed. Dietz, Scholia in Hipp. et Gal. II 205–235).

Galenos:
(p. 101) *Galeni in Hippocratis de natura hominis lib. commentarii II.*
(p. 151) *In Hippocratis vel Polybi opus de salubri victus ratione privatorum commentarius.*
Ioannes Alexandrinus (nicht Philoponus): (f. 227 b) *Scholia in Hippocratis librum de natura pueri ab ore Ioannis* (Frgm.).

Florenz, Bibl. Mediceo Laurentiana, Laurent. plut. 71, 1; s. XV.

(f. 61) *De alimento.*

Florenz, Bibl. Mediceo Laurentiana, Laurent. plut. 74, 1; s. XV.
See also **plut. [25, ?]** above.

(p. 9 b) *Iusiurandum.*
(p. 9 b) *Lex.*
(p. 10) *De arte.*
(p. 12) *De prisca medicina.*

(p. 18 b) *Praeceptiones.*
(p. 20) *De decenti ornatu.*
(p. 22) *De natura hominis.*
(p. 27 b) *De genitura.*
(p. 29 b) *De natura pueri.*
(p. 36 b) *De articulis.*
(p. 58 b) *De humoribus.*
(p. 62 b) *De ulceribus.*
(p. 66) *De morbo sacro.*
(p. 70 b) *De morbis II et III.*
(f. 70 b) *De morbis I.*
(p. 70 b) *De morbis liber IV.*
(f. 106 b) *De affectionibus.*
(p. 114 b) *De internis affectionibus.*
(p. 131 b) *De victus ratione I–III.*
(p. 150 b) *De insomniis.*
(p. 153) *De visu.*
(p. 154) *De diebus iudicatoriis.*
(p. 155) *Aphorismi.*
(p. 164) *Prognosticon.*
(p. 169 b) *De diaeta (regimine) acutorum.*
(p. 182: *De flatibus.*
(p. 185) *Vectiarius.*
(p. 190) *De ossium natura.*
(p. 193 b) *De fracturis.*
(p. 204 b) *De officina medici.*
(p. 207 b) *De mulierum affectibus.*
(p. 207) *De exsectione foetus. De exsectione pueri.*
(p. 250) *De sterilibus.*
(p. 256 b) *De superfoetatione.*
(p. 260) *De septimestri partu.*
(p. 262) *De octimestri partu.*
(p. 262 b) *De virginum morbis.*
(p. 263) *De natura muliebri.*
(p. 276) *De exsectione foetus. De exsectione pueri* (I. II).
(p. 276 b) *Praesagiorum liber I.*
(p. 276 b) *Praesagiorum liber II.*
(p. 287 b) *De fistulis.*
(p. 289 b) *De haemorroïdibus.*
(p. 290 b) *Coa praesagia.*
(p. 295 b) *De morbis popularibus I et III.*

(p. 295 b) *De morbis popularibus II, IV–VII.*
(p. 343) *Epistulae.*

Galenos: (f. 1[v]) *Linguarum sive dictionum exoletarum Hippocratis explicatio.*
Soranus: (p. 8 b) *Hippocratis genus et vita secundum Soranum.*
Erotianus, *Vocum Hippocraticarum conlectio.*

Florenz, Bibl. Mediceo Laurentiana, Laurent. plut. 74, 3; s. XII.

(p. 188 b) *Iusiurandum.*

Galenos: (p. 22) *Linguarum sive dictionum exoletarum Hippocratis explicatio.*

Florenz, Bibl. Mediceo Laurentiana, Laurent. plut. 74, 7; s. IX.

(f. 9) *De officina medici.*
(f. 13) *De fracturis.*
(f. 33[v]) *De articulis* (Inscr. Περὶ ἄρθρων ἐμβολῆς).
(f. 74) *De capitis vulneribus* (Expl. τοῦ βέλεος ἐν τῷ ὀ⟨στέῳ⟩ = L. III 246, 2).

Apollonius Citiensis: (p. 179 b) *Commentarius in Hippocratis de articulis, libri III.*
Palladius: (p. 299 b) *Scholia in Hippocratis de facturis.*
Galenos: (p. 312) *In Hippocratis de articulis librum commentarii IV.*

Florenz, Bibl. Mediceo Laurentiana, Laurent. plut. 74, 8; s. XV.

Galenos:
(p. 1) *Hippocratis aphorismi et Galeni in eos commentarii VII.*
(p. 173) *In Hippocratis prognosticum commentarii III.*

Florenz, Bibl. Mediceo Laurentiana, Laurent. plut. 74, 10; s. XIV.

(f. 13[v]) *Testamentum.*

Florenz, Bibl. Mediceo Laurentiana, Laurent. plut. 74, 11; s. XIII.

(f. 131) *Aphorismi.*
(p. 171) *Prognosticon* (»Libri III«).

Theophilus: (p. 1) *Commentarius in Hippocratis aphorismos* (Initio mutilus).

[Florenz, Bibl. Mediceo Laurentiana, Laurent. plut. 74, 12].
= plut. 74.12 (*Census*: 76, nr [0325]).

Excerpta varia.

Galenos: (p. 28 b) *Galeni in Hippocratis de natura hominis lib. commentarii II* (Frgm.).

Florenz, Bibl. Mediceo Laurentiana, Laurent. plut. 74, 13; s. XV.

(p. 5) *Aphorismi* (c. comm.).
(p. 4) *Iusiurandum.*

Soranus: (p. 3) *Hippocratis genus et vita secundum Soranum.*

Florenz, Bibl. Mediceo Laurentiana, Laurent. plut. 74, 21; s. XV.

(p. 1) *De ulceribus* (Frgm.).

Florenz, Bibl. Mediceo Laurentiana, Laurent. plut. 74, 25; s. XIV.

Galenos: (p. 127) *In Hippocratis epidemiarum libros commentarius* (in librum III).

Florenz, Bibl. Mediceo Laurentiana, Laurent. plut. 74, 31; x. XIV.

(p. 24) *De diebus iudicatoriis* (Π. κρισίμων ἡμερῶν).

Galenos: (p. 199 b) *In Hippocratis prognosticum commentarii III* (Frgm. ex libris I. II. III.).

Florenz, Bibl. Mediceo Laurentiana, Laurent. plut. 75, 3; s. XII.

Prognosticon.

Florenz, Bibl. Mediceo Laurentiana, Laurent. plut. 75, 5; s. XIV.
»*Laurent. 75, 5 + 75, 20 bilden Bd. I, 75, 18 + 75, 7 den II. Bd. derselben Aëtiushandschrift des XIV. Jahrhunderts.*« *M. W.*

Galenos:
(p. 159) *In Hippocratis librum de acutorum victu commentarii IV.*
(p. 249) *In Hippocratis prognosticum commentarii III.*

Florenz, Bibl. Mediceo Laurentiana, Laurent. plut. 75, 10; s. XV.
See also **[75, 10]** below.

(p. 1) *Prognostica* (Hipp. praenotiones quaedam et signa morborum).

[Florenz, Bibl. Mediceo Laurentiana, Laurent. plut. 75, 10; s. -].
Same as plut. **75, 10** above (*Census*: 78, nr [0354]).

Prognosticon (Hipp. praenotiones quaedam et signa morborum).

Florenz, Bibl. Mediceo Laurentiana, Laurent. plut. 75, 19; s. XIV.

(p. 16 b. 19. 20) *Excerpta varia*.

Florenz, Bibl. Mediceo Laurentiana, Laurent. plut. 75, 21; s. XIII.

Palladius: (p. 251) *Scholia in Hippocratis de popularibus morbis librum sextum, sectiones VIII* (Frgm. »Sextae et septimae sectionis fragmentum« = Dietz II p. 161, 21–171, 34. 177, 18–198, 19).

Florenz, Bibl. Mediceo Laurentiana, Laurent. plut. 75, 22; s. XV.

Palladius: (p. 1) *Scholia in Hippocratis de popularibus morbis librum sextum, sectiones VIII*.

Florenz, Bibl. Mediceo Laurentiana, Laurent. App., 2; s. XV.
= Antinori 101 (*Census*: 80, nr [0372]).

De angina.
(f. 106^{v}) *De salubri diaeta* (Frgm. Περὶ διαίτης γυναικῶν. Inc. Τὰς γυναῖκας ὧδε χρὴ διαιτᾶσθαι cf. L. VI 82, 2. Expl. καὶ τὰς σκιατραφίας cf. L. 82, 6).
(f. 222) *Jatrosophium* (Ἰατρικὸν Ἱππ. καὶ Γαλ. ἰατρεῖαι διάφοροι).
(f. 344) *De iecore*.
(f. 355) *De collo vesicae*.

Florenz, bibl. naz. [Magliabecchiana] / Magliabech.
Now Firenze, Biblioteca nazionale Magliabechiana

Florenz, bibl. naz. [Magliabecchiana], II.III.428; s. XVI.
Same as **Magliabech. 1** below.
Now *Magliabechianus* 1 (*Census*: 80, nr [0374]).

(f. 204) *De urinis* (*Wie im* Magliab. [1]. Expl. ὑφιζάνει κάτω, τοσούτῳ βελτίω γίνεται).
(f. 204) *Excerpta varia*.

Florenz, Magliabech. 1; s. XVI.
See also **bibl. naz. [Magliabecchiana], II.III.428** above.

(f. 204) *De urinis* (Inc. Οὖρον δὲ ἄριστον. Expl. τὴν ἀνωμαλίην).

Florenz, Bibl. Riccardiana
Firenze, Biblioteca Riccardiana

Florenz, Bibl. Riccardiana, Riccard. 17 (K I 24); s. XVI.
Now Riccard. 17 (*Census*: 81, nr [0378]).

Galenos: (f. 111) *In Hippocratis prognosticum commentarii III.*

Florenz, Bibl. Riccardiana, Riccard. 41 (K II 2); XVI.
Now Riccard. 41 (*Census*: 81, nr [0380]).

(f. 13) *Aphorismi* (IV 69–83 = L. IV 526–532).
(f. 13) *De urinis* (Inc. *und* expl. *wie im* Magliabecch. [1]).

Florenz, Bibl. Riccardiana, Riccard. 44 (K II 5); s. XV–XVI.
Now Riccard. 44 (*Census*: 81, nr [0381]).

(f. 1) *Aphorismi*.
(f. 13^{v}) *Prognosticon*.

Galenos:
(f. 27) *Hippocratis aphorismi et Galeni in eos commentarii VII.*
(f. 192) *In Hippocratis prognosticum commentarii III.*

Göttingen, Univ.-Bibl.
Now Göttingen, Niedersachsische Staats- und Universitätsbibliothek

Göttingen, Univ.-Bibl., Hist. nat., 3; a. 1526.
Now 4° Cod. Ms. hist. nat. 3 (*Census*: 84, nr [0388]).

Opera varia (impress. Hipp. omnia opera Venet. 1526. »Das Handexemplar des Janus Cornarius aus Zwickau ... *vgl.* Kühlewein im Hermes 27 (1892) p. 302 Anm. 3.«).

Göttingen, Univ.-Bibl., Hist. nat., 4; a. 1538.
Now 4° Cod. Ms. hist. nat. 4 (*Census*: 85, nr [0389]).

Opera varia (Impress. Hipp. libri omnes Basil. 1538. »Handexemplar des Joh. Opsopoeus ... *vgl.* Kühlewein, Hermes 27 (1892) p. 303«).

Göttingen, Univ.-Bibl., Hist. nat., 5; s. XVII.
Now 4° Cod. Ms. hist. nat. 5 (*Census*: 84, nr [0390]).

Theophilus, *Commentarius in Hippocratis aphorismos.*

Göttingen, Univ.-Bibl., Philol., 2; s. XVIII.
Now 8° Cod. Ms. philol. 2 (*Census*: 84, nr [0393]).

(f. 89) *De remediis* (»ex manuscr. Hadriani Junii Hornani«).

Göttingen, Univ.-Bibl., Philol., 21; s. XVII–XVIII.
Now 8° Cod. Ms. philol. 21 (*Census*: 84, nr [0394]).

(f. 77) *De remediis* (»ex manuscr. Hadr. Iun. Hornani miss. ex Anglia a Rich. Thomone«).

Heidelberg, Bibl. Univ.
Now Heidelberg, Universitätsbibliothek

Heidelberg, Bibl. Univ., 132; s. XV.
= Cod. Pal. graec. 132 (*Census*: 88, nr [0399]).

(nr 14) *Epistulae.*

Heidelberg, Bibl. Univ., 155; s. XV.
= Cod. Pal. graec. 155 (*Census*: 88, nr [0400]).

(nr 4) *Epistula ad Ptolemaeum regem de sanitate tuenda.*

Heidelberg, Bibl. Univ., 398; s. X.
= Cod. Pal. graec. 398 (*Census*: 89, nr [0402]).

(nr 16) *Epistulae.*

Holkham

Holkham, Bibl. des Gr. Leicester, 282; s. XVI.
Now Oxford, Bodleian Library, MS. Holkham Gr. 92 (*Census*: 89, nr [0403]).
See also [**Padua, Bibl. Canonicor. Lateranens.**] (p. 54), and **Padua, Bibl. S. Joannis in Viridario, ad dextr. plut. XVII** (p. 54) below.

(nr 2) *Aphorismi* (Expl. καὶ σαρκὶ παρέδωκεν).
(nr 3) *Prognosticon.*
(nr 4) *De diaeta (regimine) acutorum* (Inscr. ἱππ. πρὸς τὰς κνιδίας γνώμας ἢ περὶ πτισάνης).
(nr 5) *De officina medici.*
(nr 6) *De fracturis.*
(nr 7) *De articulis.*
(nr 8) *De capitis vulneribus.*
(nr 9) *De aëre, aquis et locis.*
(nr 10) *De morbis popularibus I et III.*
(nr 10) *De morbis popularibus II. IV–VII.*
(nr 11) *De febribus.*
(nr 11) *De natura hominis.*
(nr 11) *De salubri diaeta.*
(nr 12) *De natura pueri.*
(nr 13) *De genitura* (Expl. ἐν τῇσι μήτρῃσιν τῆς γυναικός).
(nr 14) *De septimestri partu* (Inc. Περὶ δὲ ἑπταμήνων ὁ λόγος. Expl. ταῦτα οὖν πρότερον ἐννοούμενος).
(nr 15) *De octimestri partu* (Inc. Φημὶ δισσὰς ἐφεξῆς κακοπαθείας γιγνομένας. Expl. ἄρχονται ἐν τούτῳ τῷ χρόνῳ).
(nr 16) *De locis in homine.*
(nr 17) *De medico.*
(nr 18) *De iudicationibus.*
(nr 18[a]) *De corde.*
(nr 18[b]) *De carnibus.*

(nr 19) *De glandulis.*
(nr 20) *De anatome.*
(nr 21) *De virginum morbis.*
(nr 22) *De natura muliebri.*
(nr 23) *De dentitione.*
(nr 24 *und* 25) *De mulierum affectibus.*
(nr 26 *und* 27) *De exsectione foetus. De exsectione pueri* (I. II).

Holkham, Bibl. des Gr. Leicester, 293; s.
Now Oxford, Bodleian Library, MS. Holkham Gr. 106 (*Census*: 90, nr [0406]).

Aphorismi.

Jerusalem, Bibl. d. hl. Grabes
Now at Αθήνα, Εθνική Βιβλιοθήκη της Ελλάδος ΕΒΕ, Μετόχιον Παναγίου Τάφου–ΜΠΤ

Jerusalem, Bibl. d. hl. Grabes, 189; s. XVIII.
Now ΜΠΤ 189 (*Census*: 92, nr [0411] and p. 15).

(f. 299) *De septimanis* (Frgm. 229 ? Ἑπτὰ ἡλικίαι τῶν ἀνθρ.).

Jerusalem, Bibl. Mar-Saba
Ιερουσαλήμ, Πατριαρχείο, Ιερά Μονή Αγίου Σάββα

Jerusalem, Bibl. Mar-Saba, 432; a. 1662.
= Ιερά Μονή Αγίου Σάββα, 432 (*Census*: 93, nr [0421]).

Hippokrates, **Galenos**, **Meletius monachus**: (f. 1) *Jatrosophium* (Ἰατροσόφιον ... Γαλ. Ἱππ. καὶ Μελετίου).

Jerusalem, Bibl. Mar-Saba, 481; s. XVIII.
= Ιερά Μονή Αγίου Σάββα, 481 (*Census*: 93, nr [0422]).

(f. 265) *Aphorismi* (Μετάφρασις τῶν ἀφ. τοῦ Ἱππ. εἰς τὴν κοινὴν διάλεκτον ... ἐκ τῆς τοῦ Γαλ. διδασκαλίας).

Galenos: (f. 265) *Hippocratis aphorismi et Galeni in eos commentarii VII* (Μετάφρασις τῶν ἀφ. τοῦ Ἱππ. εἰς τὴν κοινὴν διάλεκτον ... ἐκ τῆς τοῦ Γαλ. διδασκαλίας).

Jerusalem, Bibl. Mar-Saba, 498; s. XVIII.
= Ιερά Μονή Αγίου Σάββα, 498 (*Census*: 93, nr [0423]).

(f. 1) *Aphorismi*.
(f. 25) *Prognosticon* (Ἐξήγησις τῶν προγνωστικῶν Ἱππ.).
(f. 37) *Praesagiorum liber I* (Ἱππ. προρρητικῶν ἐξήγησις).
(f. 37) *Praesagiorum liber II* (Ἱππ. προρρητικῶν ἐξήγησις).

Jerusalem, Bibl. patriarch.
Ιερουσαλήμ, Πατριαρχείο, Πανάγιος Τάφος

Jerusalem, Bibl. patriarch., 102; s. XVIII.
= Πανάγιος Τάφος, 102 (*Census* 94, nr [0425]).

(f. 1) *Opera varia* (»Συγγράμματα Ἱππ.«).
(f. 12) *Aphorismi* (Ἑρμηνεία εἰς τοὺς ἀφ. Ἱππ., καταστρωθεῖσα εἰς κοινὴν φράσιν παρὰ Μπαλάνου Βασιλοπούλου κτλ.).

Galenos: (f. 12) *Hippocratis aphorismi et Galeni in eos commentarii VII* (Ἑρμηνεία εἰς τοὺς ἀφ. Ἱππ., καταστρωθεῖσα εἰς κοινὴν φράσιν παρὰ Μπαλάνου Βασιλοπούλου ... κατὰ τὸν Γαληνόν).

Jerusalem, Bibl. patriarch., 148; s. XVI.
= Πανάγιος Τάφος, 148 (*Census* 94, nr [0427]).

(f. 15v) *Jatrosophium*.

Jerusalem, Bibl. patriarch., 463; s. XVIII.
= Πανάγιος Τάφος, 463 (*Census* 94, nr [0431]).

(nr 8) *Excerpta varia*.

Karlsruhe, Großherzogl. Hof. u. Landesbibliothek
Now Badische Landesbibliothek Karlsruhe

Karlsruhe, Großherzogl. Hof. u. Landesbibliothek, 449, s. XV/XVI, XV–XVI.
Now K 449 (*Census*: 95, nr [0434]).

De genitura.
De natura pueri (fine mutil.).

(f. 1) *Aphorismi* (Sectio III–VII).
(f. 62–73^v) *De diaeta (regimine) acutorum* (= Kühn Med. Gr. Op. XXII p. 26–36. Initium deest).

Kopenhagen, Königl. Bibliothek.
Now København, Det Kongelige Bibliotek

Kopenhagen, Königl. Bibliothek, Hauniens. ant. fund. reg. 224; s. XVI.
Now GkS 224, 2° (*Census*: 102, nr [0445]).

Coa praesagia.
De affectionibus.
De alimento.
De arte.
De articulis.
De decenti ornatu.
De diaeta (regimine) acutorum.
De diebus iudicatoriis.
De exsectione foetus. De exsectione pueri (I. II).
De fistulis.
De flatibus.
De fracturis.
De genitura.
De haemorroïdibus.
De humoribus.
De insomniis.
De internis affectionibus.
De morbis I.
De morbis II et III.
De morbis liber IV.
De morbis popularibus I et III.
De morbis popularibus II. IV–VII.
De morbo sacro.
De mulieribus.
De mulierum affectibus.
De natura hominis.
De natura muliebri.
De officina medici.
De natura pueri.
De octimestri partu.

De ossium natura.
De prisca medicina.
De salubri diaeta.
De septimestri partu.
De sterilibus.
De superfoetatione.
De ulceribus.
De victus ratione I–III.
De virginum morbis.
De visu.
Epistulae (Expl. μακρῶν μεγάλοι προσεδεήθησαν = L. IX 424, 16).
Iusiurandum (Sequitur ἕτερος ὅρκος Ἱπποκράτους. Inc. Αὐτὸν ἐν ἀχράντοισι. Expl. ὀλβιόδωρον ὑγείην = Hipp. I 74 Kuehlew. *Vgl.* Kuehn, *Additam. ad Fabricii elenchum medicorum vet.* XV. [Lips. 1828] p. 11).
Lex.
Praesagiorum liber I.
Praesagiorum liber II.
Praeceptiones.
Prognosticon.
Vectiarius.

Galenos, *Linguarum sive dictionum exoletarum Hippocratis explicatio. Aphorismi.*
Soranus, *Hippocratis genus et vita secundum Soranum.*

Leipzig, Universitätsbibliothek
Now Leipzig, Universitätsbibliothek «Bibliotheca Albertina»

Leipzig, Universitätsbibliothek, 56; s. XIX.
= Cod. graec. 56 (*Census*: 107, nr [0460]).

Galenos, *In Hippocratis de humoribus librum commentarii III.*

Leipzig, Universitätsbibliothek, 59; s. XIX.
= Cod. graec. 59 (*Census*: 107, nr [0463]).

Apollonius Citiensis: (nr 2) *Commentarius in Hippocratis de articulis, libri III* (conscr. a Fr. del Furia Florentino et a K. G. Kuehnio).

Leipzig, Universitätsbibliothek, 61; s. XIX.
= Cod. graec. 61 (*Census*: 107, nr [0465]).

Opera varia (»Lectiones cod. Hauniensis 224 in folio, qui Hipp. opera continet collata cum editione C. G. Kuehnii verglichen von O. D. Bloch Kopenhagen 1825. Vorn ein halbes Blatt in zwei Kolumnen geschrieben: ‚Ex editione Van der Linden. Observ. crit. a Coraës mihi missae.' Am Schlusse zwei Blätter mit einer Abschrift des cod. 109 (Bl. 6), geschrieben von F. Jacobs, München 2. Aug. 1818«).

Leipzig, Universitätsbibliothek, 64; s. XVIII.
= Cod. graec. 64 (*Census*: 108, nr [0468]).

Apollonius Citiensis: (p. 1) *Commentarius in Hippocratis de articulis, libri III.*

Lesbos, Βιβλ. τῆς τοῦ Λειμῶνος Μονῆς
Now Καλλονή Λέσβου, Βιβλιοθήκη τῆς τοῦ Λειμῶνος Μονῆς

Lesbos, Βιβλ. τῆς τοῦ Λειμῶνος Μονῆς, 175; s. XVII.
Καλλονή Λέσβου, Βιβλιοθήκη τῆς τοῦ Λειμῶνος Μονῆς, 175.

Excerpta varia.

Leyden, Universitäts-Bibliothek
Now Leiden, Universiteitsbibliotheek

Leyden, Universitäts-Bibliothek, B. P., 670; s. XVI.
= Bibliotheca Publica Graeca 67 Octavo (now BPG 67 O) (*Census*: 109, nr [0479]).

Opera varia (»Handschriftl. Bemerkungen des Vulcanius, wie es scheint«).

Leyden, Universitäts-Bibliothek, Scal. 71; s. XVI.
= *Scaligerianus* 71 (now SCA 71) (*Census*: 110, nr [0484]).

(f. 1) *Aphorismi.*
(f. 57–91) *Prognosticon.*
(f. 92) *Excerpta varia* (Περὶ τῆς ᾗ χρῆται Ἱπποκράτης διαλέκτου. Sunt 17 regulae grammaticae).

Leyden, Universitäts-Bibliothek, Voss. 4° 38; s. XV.
= *Vossianus graecus* in quarto 38 (now VGQ 38) (*Census*: 113, nr [0499]).

Epistulae (Ep. 17).

Leyden, Universitäts-Bibliothek, Voss. 4° 50; s. XV.
= *Vossianus graecus* in quarto 50 (now VGQ 50) (*Census*: 113, nr [0501]).

Hippiatrica (Ἱππιατρ. τοῦ σοφοῦ ῥήτορος Ἱερακλέου καὶ Ἱππ. κ. τοῦ σοφ. Γαλ.).

Leyden, Universitäts-Bibliothek, Voss. 8° 7; XVII.
= *Vossianus graecus* in octavo 7 (now VGO 7) (*Census*: 113, nr [0503]).

De remediis (descr. Is. Vossius ex Hadr. Iun. Hornani msto.).

Leyden, Universitäts-Bibliothek, Voss. fol. 10; s. XVI.
= *Vossianus graecus* in folio 10 (now VGF 10) (*Census*: 113, nr [0506]).

Coa praesagia.
De affectionibus.
De alimento.
De arte.
De articulis.
De diaeta (regimine) acutorum.
De decenti ornatu.
De diebus iudicatoriis.
De exsectione foetus. De exsectione pueri (I. II).
De febribus (Inc. Οἱ πλεῖστοι τῶν πυρετῶν).
De fistulis.
De flatibus.
De fracturis.
De haemorroïdibus.
De humoribus.
De insomniis.
De morbo sacro.
De morbis popularibus I et III.
De morbis popularibus II. IV–VII.
De mulierum affectibus.
De natura hominis.
De natura muliebri.
De natura pueri.
De ossium natura.
De prisca medicina.

De salubri diaeta.
De specie atrae bilis.
De sterilibus.
De substantia artis medicae. Definitio artis medicae.
De superfoetatione.
De ulceribus.
De urinis.
De victus ratione I–III.
De visu.
Esse re vera artes.
Iusiurandum.
Lex.
Prognosticon.
Vectiarius.

Soranus, *Hippocratis genus et vita secundum Soranum* (*Vgl.* Hipp. Ed. Ermerins prf. p. IX).

Leyden, Universitäts-Bibliothek, Voss. Miscell. 1 pars 13; s. XV.
= *Vossianus miscellaneus* 1 (now VMI 1) (*Census*: 114–115, nr [0517]).

Galenos, *Linguarum sive dictionum exoletarum Hippocratis explicatio.*

Leyden, Universitäts-Bibliothek, Vulc. 56; s. XIV.
= *Vulcanianus* 56 (now VUL 56) (*Census*: 115, nr [0521]).

(f. 131–133) *Ad Ptolemaeum regem epistula de hominis fabrica.*

Leyden, Universitäts-Bibliothek, Vulc. 108 pars 15; s. XVI.
= *Vulcanianus* 108 (now VUL 108) (*Census*: 115, nr [0523]).

De remediis (Frgm.).

London, British Museum
Now London, British Library

London, British Museum, Addit. 6898; s. XIII (XIV), XIII/XIV.

(f. 160^{v}) *Aphorismi* (c. scholiis; Inc. ⟨ἐπε⟩ιδή⟨π⟩ερ ἐνταῦθα σκοπὸν ἔχει ὁ Γαληνός).

London, British Museum, Addit. 28, 830; s. XVII.

(f. 15) *Jatrosophium* (Ἰατροσόφ. ... Ἱππ. καὶ Γαλ. Inc. Παρὶ τῆς πεγουνέας [sic]).

London, British Museum, Addit. 34,060; s. XV.

(f. 481) *Epistula ad Ptolemaeum regem de sanitate tuenda* (Expl. τοῖς δὲ μείζοσιν ἐνεργεστέρας).

London, British Museum, Arundel. 538; s. XV.

(f. 1) *Aphorismi.*
(f. 19) *Iusiurandum.*
(f. 21) *De natura pueri.*
(f. 45) *De genitura.*
(f. 53ᵛ) *Lex.*
(f. 55–56) *De arte* (Expl. f. 56 δυνάμενος διὰ σοφίην ἢ πεπαίδευται = VI 2, 18 L.).

London, British Museum, Harleian. 5611; s. XV.

Galenos: (f. 1) *Hippocratis aphorismi et Galeni in eos commentarii VII.*

London, British Museum, Harleian. 5626; s. XV (XVI), XV (XVI ?), XV–XVI, XV–XVI (?).

(f. 2) **Hippokrates, Galenos,** *Jatrosophium* (Ἰατροσόφ. ... Ἱππ. καὶ Γαλ. κτλ.).
(f. 80) *Epistula ad Ptolemaeum regem de sanitate tuenda* (Expl. ἔπειτα θερμάνας ἄλειφε καὶ δῆσον).
(f. 86) *Aphorismi* (Libri II–VI. L. IV 470–576,1; Expl. τοῖσι σπληνώδεσι δυσεντερίη γενομένη ἀγαθόν).

London, British Museum, Harleian. 5635; s. XV.

(f. 128ᵛ) *Epistulae* (Ep. 17).
(f. 227ᵛ) *Epistulae* (Ep. 1; des. haec series f. 229 νούσων παύειν, ἐχθροὺς ἐόντας Ἑλλήνων = Expl. *Epistulae* 5).

London, British Museum, Harleian. 6295; s. XV (XIV sec. catal.), XV (XIV).

(f. 89) *Prognosticon.*
(f. 103) *De febrium differentiis* (Inc. πυρετοί · οἱ μὲν δακνώδεις εἰσί. Expl. ἐν οἷς αἱ διαφοραὶ τῶν πυρετῶν).
(f. 106) *Epistula ad Ptolemaeum regem de sanitate tuenda* (Expl. εἰσὶ μόνον, ἀλλὰ καὶ ἔξω).
(f. 157) *Aphorismi* (c. comm. pleniore).

London, British Museum, Harleian. 6301; s. XV, XVI.

(f. 3ᵛ) *Epistulae* (3–9).

London, British Museum, Regius 16. C. XVI; s. XVI.
Now Royal. 16.C.xvi.

(f. 48) *Prognosticon*.

London, British Museum, Stowe 1073; s. XVI.

(f. 2) *Iusiurandum*.
(f. 3ᵛ) *Lex*.
(f. 6) *Aphorismi* (Expl. χολῇ καὶ αἵματι καὶ φλέγματι καὶ σαρκὶ παρέδωκεν).
(f. 62ᵛ) *Prognosticon*.

London, Medical Society
Now at the Wellcome Library, London

London, Medical Society, AA a 1 = Xa 32; s. XVI.
Now London, Wellcome Library, MS. MSL 14 (*Census*: 121, nr [0562]).

(p. 1) *Ad Ptolemaeum regem epistula de hominis fabrica* (Expl. συνάγεται ὁ ἐνιαυτὸς εἰς ἡμέρας τξε'; *Vgl.* Athos Ἰβήρ. 5034. 914.).
(p. 12) *De corpore et generatione hominis* (Inc. Ἀλλὰ μηδεὶς ὑπολαμβανέτω παντελῶς ἄψυχον εἶναι τὴν γονήν. Expl. κομάτια καὶ μέρη, διακόσια εἴκοσι ἐννέα).
(p. 34) *Sententiae de vita et morte* (Inc. Ὁ ἐμπειρικώτατος ἁπάντων. Expl. εἰς κ' ἡμέρας ἀποθανεῖται).

London, Medical Society, HHi 17 = We 30; s. XV in.
Now London, Wellcome Library, MS. MSL 60 (*Census*: 121, nr [0564]).

(f. 1) *Aphorismi*.
(f. 12) *Prognosticon*.
(nr 21 Dbg.) *Remedia*.

London, Medical Society, HH i 21. 22 = We 28. 29; s. XV.
Now London, Wellcome Library, MS. MSL 52 A&B (*Census*: 121, nr [0565]).

(f. 361ᵛ) *Sententiae de vita et morte* (Inc. und Expl. wie im Lond. [Medical Society] AA a 1) (p. 35).

Madrid, Nationalbibliothek
Madrid, Biblioteca Nacional

Madrid, Nationalbibliothek, 4557 (N 119); s. XV ex.
= 4557 (*Census*: 125, nr [0575]).

(f. 94–124) *Epistulae*.

Madrid, Nationalbibliothek, 4634 (olim N 112); s. XV.
= 4634 (*Census*: 125, nr [0580]).

(f. 2) *Aphorismi*.
(f. 36) *Prognosticon*.

Mailand, Bibl. Ambrosiana
Milano, Biblioteca Ambrosiana

Mailand, Bibl. Ambrosiana, A 45 Sup.; s. XIII.

(f. 50) *Ad Ptolemaeum regem epistula de hominis fabrica* (Expl. συνάγεται ὁ ἐνιαυτὸς εἰς ἡμέρας τξε').
(f. 61ᵛ) *Epistula ad Ptolemaeum regem de sanitate tuenda* (Expl. ἐκ τῆς προσθήκης τῶν ια' ἡμερῶν).

Mailand, Bibl. Ambrosiana, A 95 Sup.; s. XV.

(f. 4) *Sententiae de vita et morte* (Inc. *und* Expl. *wie im* Lond. Medical Society [AA a 1 = Xa 32]) (above p. 35).
(f. 95) *Ad Ptolemaeum regem epistula de hominis fabrica*.

Theophilus: (f. 165) *Commentarius in Hippocratis aphorismos* (= »Dietz II 245 sub finem, 247, 7–300,15 passim«).

Mailand, Bibl. Ambrosiana, A 110 Sup.; s. XV–XVI.

(f. 60ᵛ) *Epistula ad Ptolemaeum regem de sanitate tuenda*.

Mailand, Bibl. Ambrosiana, A 156 Sup.; s. XVI.

(f. 1) *Aphorismi* (Expl. πάνυ πολλὴ θανάσιμος).
(f. 13) *Prognosticon*.

(f. 20) *Praesagiorum liber I.*

Galenos:
(f. 24) *Hippocratis aphorismi et Galeni in eos commentarii VII.*
(f. 190) *In Hippocratis prognosticum commentarii III.*

Mailand, Bibl. Ambrosiana, B 72 Sup.; s. –.
s. XV.

(f. 116) *Hippocratis ad Ptolemaeum regem epistula.*
(f. 116^{v}) *Ad Ptolemaeum regem epistula de hominis fabrica* (Expl. ὑγιεῖ δ' ἔσονται).

Mailand, Bibl. Ambrosiana, B 108 Sup.; s. XIV in.

(f. 1) *De natura muliebri* (L. VII 318, 11–370, 11. 386, 3–416, 12).
(f. 12) *Praesagiorum liber II* (Inc. = L. IX 12, 16).
(f. 19) *De victus ratione I–III* (Libri I. II).

Mailand, Bibl. Ambrosiana, B 113 Sup.; s. XIV in.

(f. 1) *Lex.*
(f. 1) *Qualem oporteat esse discipulum* (Inc. Δεῖ εἶναι. Expl. ἰητρῷ ἁρμοδιώτερον).
(f. 2) *Iusiurandum.*
(f. 171^{v}) *Prognosticon.*
(f. 181) *De flatibus* (Inscr. ἐκ τοῦ π. φύσεων).
(f. 181^{v}) *De remediis* (Frgm. Inc. Τὰ δὲ περὶ φαρμάκων πρήγματα. Expl. τῶν παραπλησίων).
(f. 184) *Epistulae.*
(f. 203^{v}) *Iusiurandum* (Inscr. wie im Bonon. 3632 [p. 12]. »Textus hac forma ✝ scriptus«).

Theophilus: (f. 4) *Commentarius in Hippocratis aphorismos* (= Dietz II 245–543).
Palladius: (f. 85) *Scholia in Hippocratis de popularibus morbis librum sextum, sectiones VIII.*

Mailand, Bibl. Ambrosiana, B 126 Sup.; s. XIV, XIV ex.

(f. 166) *De affectionibus.*

Mailand, Bibl. Ambrosiana, C 4 Sup.; s. –, XV.

(f. 244^{v}) *De venae sectione.*

Mailand, Bibl. Ambrosiana, C 85 Sup.; s. XV–XVI.

De alimento.
De diebus iudicatoriis.
De exsectione foetus. De exsectione pueri.
De flatibus (»De naturis«; vielmehr Excerpt aus π. φυσῶν verm. Schoene).
De fracturis.
De humoribus.
De insomniis.
De morbis I.
De morbis II et III.
De morbis liber IV.
De morbo sacro.
De mulierum affectibus.
De natura muliebri.
De octimestri partu.
De ossium natura.
De septimestri partu.
De sterilibus.
De superfoetatione.
De ulceribus.
De victus ratione I–III.
De virginum morbis.
Vectiarius.

Mailand, Bibl. Ambrosiana, C 118 Sup.; s. –.
Ambros. muß heißen C 119 Sup.; s. XVI.
See **C 119 Sup.** below.

Galenos, *In Hippocratis de humoribus librum commentarii III* (non sine lacunis, ut videtur).

Mailand, Bibl. Ambrosiana, C 119 Sup.; s. XV.
= L 119 sup. and not C 119 sup.
= L 119 sup. (*Census*: 131, nr [0620]). See also **C 118 Sup.** above.

Galenos, *In Hippocratis de humoribus librum commentarii III.*

Mailand, Bibl. Ambrosiana, F 23 Sup.; s. XV.

(f. 131^{v}) *Excerpta varia* (Διαίρεσις ἀνθρώπου. Inc. Διαιροῦμεν δὲ τὸν ἄνθρωπον. Expl. ἐξόχως ἐνταῦθα γενησόμενα).

(f. 219^{v}) *Ad Ptolemaeum regem epistula de hominis fabrica* (Inc. Ἀλλὰ μὴ ὑπολαμβάνῃς. Expl. ἐν τοῖς ἀριστεροῖς θύλη).

(f. 222) *Excerpta varia* (Inscr. Περὶ καταστάσεως ἀνθρώπου. Inc. Συνέστηκεν δὲ ὁ ἄνθρωπος ἐκ τινῶν, ἤγουν. Expl. φαντασία καὶ αἰσθήσεις).

Mailand, Bibl. Ambrosiana, L 30 Sup.; a. 1524.

Theophilus: (f. 1) *Commentarius in Hippocratis aphorismos* (= Dietz II 245–543, 4. »Falso Philotheus pro Theophilo scriptum est«).

Stephanus Alexandrinus: (f. 127) *Scholia in Hippocratis praenotiones. Sectiones III.*

Mailand, Bibl. Ambrosiana, L 110 Sup.; s. XVI.

(f. 30) *De morbo sacro.*
(f. 233^{v}) *Lex.*
(f. 234) *De arte.*
(f. 241^{v}) *De natura hominis.*
(f. 244^{v}) *De salubri diaeta.*
(f. 235^{v}) *De prisca medicina.*
(f. 240^{v}) *De decenti ornatu.*
(f. 239^{v}) *Praeceptiones.*
(f. 245^{v}) *De genitura.*
(f. 246^{v}) *De natura pueri.*
(f. 251^{v}) *De articulis.*
(f. 270) *De humoribus.*
(f. 272^{v}) *De alimento.*
(f. 274) *De ulceribus.*
(f. 282^{v}) *De morbis II et III.*
(f. 282^{v}) *De morbis I.*
(f. 282^{v}) *De morbis liber IV.*
(f. 324) *De affectionibus* (mutil.).

Theophilus: (f. 1) *Commentarius in Hippocratis aphorismos* (»In prooemio non semper verba eadem atque apud Dietz II 245«).

Soranus: (f. 233) *Hippocratis genus et vita secundum Soranum.*

Mailand, Bibl. Ambrosiana, P 90 Sup.; s. XV–XVI.

(f. 79^{v}) *Prognosticon* (»Dialecto communi scripta«).

Mailand, Bibl. Ambrosiana, Q 3 Sup.; s. XV–XVI.

Galenos: (f. 129) *In Hippocratis praedictionum librum primum commentarii III.*

Mailand, Bibl. Ambrosiana, Q 13 Sup.; s. –.
s. XV–XVI.

(f. 4) *Prognosticon* (Frgm. Inc. ἢ ὁ ἕτερος τοῦ ἑτέρου. Expl. ἐπιγενομένων σημείων).

Mailand, Bibl. Ambrosiana, S 19 Sup.; s. –.

Stephanus Atheniensis, **Theophilus**, *In aphorismos Hippocratis commentarius/Commentarius in Hippocratis aphorismos* (»Stephani et Theoph. in aphor. Hipp. comm.«).

Mailand, Bibl. Ambrosiana, T 19 Sup.; s. –.
s. XV.

Aphorismi.

Mailand, Bibl. Ambrosiana, A 27 Inf.; s. XVI.

Stephanus Alexandrinus: (f. 2) *Scholia in Hippocratis praenotiones. Sectiones III* (»Operi sine auctoris nomine tradito praemittitur poëma«).

Mailand, Bibl. Ambrosiana, H 2 Inf.; s. XVI.

(f. 240v) *Sententiae de vita et morte.*
(f. 268) *De partibus hominis* (Inc. Βρέγμα τὸ λεγόμενον ἁπαλόν).

Mailand, Bibl. Ambrosiana, S. Q. E. VIII 13.
= S.Q.E.VIII.13 (*Census*: 136, nr [0676]).

(f. 6–30v) *Opera varia* (Handschriftliche Bemerkungen aus Aldina Edition).

Mailand, Bibl. Ambrosiana, S.Q.T.VIII 9.
= S.Q.T.VIII.9 (*Census*: 136, nr [0679]).

De aëre, aquis et locis (Ed. Basil. mit Randbemerkungen zu π. ἀέρων etc.).

Mailand, Bibliotheca Trivulziana
Now Milano, Archivio Storico Civico e Biblioteca Trivulziana

Mailand, Bibl. Trivulziana, 685, s. XIV, XV (XIV).
Milano, Archivio Storico Civico e Biblioteca Trivulziana, 685.

Galenos:
(f. 120) *In Hippocratis librum de acutorum victu commentarii IV*.
(f. 122ᵛ–193) *In Hippocratis librum de acutorum victu commentarii IV*.
(f. 193–230) *In Hippocratis praedictionum librum primum commentarii III* (Libri I et II; lib. II inc. ἂν ᾖ κατὰ μὲν τὴν χρόαν, ὕπωχρον μετρίως = K. XVI 588, 14; expl. ἢ σπόνδυλος ἐγκάθηται, τουτέοισιν = K. 678).

Modena, Bibl. Estense
Now Modena, Biblioteca Estense Universitaria

Modena, Bibl. Estense, 54 (III B 2); s. XV.
Now α.U.9.3 (*Census*: 141, nr [0688]).

(f. 121) *Epistulae* (1–5. 11–17 usque ad ὠχριακῶς πάνυ).

Modena, Bibl. Estense, 61 (III B 9); s. XV.
Now α.U.9.4 (*Census*: 141, nr [0689]).

(f. 29ᵛ) *Iusiurandum*.
(f. 31) *Excerpta varia*.

Modena, Bibl. Estense, 85 (III C 6); s. XV.
Now α.Q.5.16 (*Census*: 141, nr [0691]).

(f. 95) *De IV aetatibus praenotio* (Inc. Ἂν μὲν χειμὼν αὐχμηρός. Expl. κόρυζαι χρόνιαι, ἐνίοισι δὲ καὶ μελαγχολίαι).
(f. 95ᵛ) *Prognostica* (Πρόγνωσις π. τῶν δ' ὡρῶν. Inc. Ἂν μὲν χειμὼν αὐχμηρός. Expl. καὶ μελαγχολίαι).

Modena, Bibl. Estense, 115 (II D 16); s. XV.
Now α.P.5.17 (*Census*: 141, nr [0695]).

(f. 12) *Ad Ptolemaeum regem epistula de hominis fabrica*.

Modena, Bibl. Estense, 191; s. XV.
Now α.N.8.8 (*Census*: 142, nr [0701]).

Epistulae (1–5. 11–18. 20).

Modena, Bibl. Estense, 211 (III G 7); s. XV.
Now α.G.3.11 (*Census*: 142, nr [0703]).

Galenos, *In Hippocratis epidemiarum libros commentarii* (in Hipp. de morb. popul. Lib. I et III).

Modena, Bibl. Estense, 213 (III G 9); s. XV.
Now α.G.3.12 (*Census*: 142, nr [0705]).

(f. 235) *De salubri diaeta* (Frgm. Inc. *und* Expl. *wie im* [Florent.] Laurent. App. 2) (p. 23).

Modena, Bibl. Estense, 218 (II H 3); s. XVI.
Now α.O.4.6 (*Census*: 142, nr [0708]).

(f. 110^{v}) *De genitura*.

Modena, Bibl. Estense, 220 (II H 5); s. XV.
Now α.O.4.8 (*Census*: 142, nr [0710]).

(f. 2) *De humoribus*.
(f. 6) *De alimento*.
(f. 8) *De ulceribus*.
(f. 14) *De morbo sacro*.
(f. 21) *De morbis I*.
(f. 21^{v}) *De morbis II et III*.
(f. 63^{v}) *De aëre, aquis et locis*.
(f. 71) *De morbis liber IV*.
(f. 86^{v}) *De affectionibus*.
(f. 100^{v}) *De internis affectionibus*.
(f. 129^{v}) *De victus ratione I–III*.
(f. 164) *De insomniis*.
(f. 168^{v}) *De visu*.
(f. 169^{v}) *De diebus iudicatoriis*.

Modena, Bibl. Estense, 227 (II H 12); s. XVI.
Now α.O.4.14 (*Census*: 142, nr [0712]).

(f. 3) *De flatibus*.

(f. 7v) *De ossium natura.*
(f. 21) *De fracturis.*
(f. 39v) *De officina medici.*
(f. 42) *De exsectione foetus. De exsectione pueri.*
(f. 44) *De mulierum affectibus.*
(f. 115v) *De sterilibus.*
(f. 128) *De superfoetatione.*
(f. 134) *De septimestri partu.*
(f. 137v) *De octimestri partu.*
(f. 139) *De virginum morbis.*
(f. 139v) *De natura muliebri.*
(f. 163) *De exsectione foetus. De exsectione pueri* (I. II).
(f. 164) *De fistulis.*
(f. 167) *De haemorroïdibus.*

Modena, Bibl. Estense, 233 (III H 5); s. XV.
Now α.T.1.12 (*Census*: 142, nr [0713]).

(f. 33) *De morbis popularibus I et III.*
(f. 13) *Aphorismi.*
(f. 33) *De morbis popularibus II. IV–VII.*
(f. 127) *De natura hominis.*
(f. 139v) *De genitura.*
(f. 144) *De natura pueri.*
(f. 159v) *De articulis.*

Modena, Bibl. Estense, 237 (III G 18); s. XVI.
Now α.W.3.12 (*Census*: 143, nr [0714]).

Galenos:
(f. 3) *In Hippocratis praedictionum librum primum commentarii III.*
(f. 93) *In Hippocratis prognosticum commentarii III.*

Modena, Bibl. Estense, 240 (III F 17); s. XV–XVI.
Now α.J.6.28 (*Census*: 142, nr [0715]).

Galenos: (f. 8) *Galeni in Hippocratis de natura hominis lib. commentarii II* (Expl. τὰ περὶ τὴν γῆν · οὐ μὴν κεκραμένον γε = K. XV 50, 3; Expl.: κεκραμένων [sic recte] γε.).

Moskau, Synodialbibl.
Now Государственный Исторический Музей (ГИМ), Синодальная Библиотека Московского Патриархата (Gosudarstvennyi Istoricheskii Muzei [GIM], Sinodal'naia Biblioteka Moskovskogo Patriarchata [State Historical Museum [GIM], Synodial Library of Moscow Patriarchate])

[Moskau, Synodialbibl., ?].
Now Jena, Thüringer Universitäts- und Landesbibliothek, Ms. G.B. f. 31 (*Census*: 145, nr [0719]).

Galenos, *Linguarum sive dictionum exoletarum Hippocratis explicatio.*

Moskau, Synodialbibl., 439; s. XVI.
Now Sinod. 426 (*Census*: 147, nr [0729]).

(f. 128) *Ad Ptolemaeum regem epistula de hominis fabrica.*
(f. 128) *Epistula ad Ptolemaeum regem de sanitate tuenda.*

Moskau, Synodialbibl., 465; s. XV.
Now Sinod. 282 (*Census*: 147, nr [0732]).

Galenos: (f. 33) *In Hippocratis librum de acutorum victu commentarii IV* (Libri I et III).

Moskau, Synodialbibl., 466; s. XVI.
= Sinod. 283 (*Census*: 147, nr [0733]).

Galenos : (f. 61–63) *In Hippocratis de humoribus librum commentarii III* (Auctoris nomen deest et discrepat initium; Inc. Χυμοὶ καθ' Ἱππ. εἰσὶ ...; in fine mutil.).
Stephanus Alexandrinus: (f. 89) *Scholia in Hippocratis de facturis.*
Galenos: (f. 90) *In Hippocratis librum de fracturis commentarii III* (discrepat init.).

München, Hof- und Staatsbibliothek
Now München, Bayerische Staatsbibliothek

München, Hof- und Staatsbibliothek, graec. 71; a. 1531.

(f. 11) *Iusiurandum.*
De aëre, aquis et locis.
De prisca medicina.
Prognosticon.
De diaeta (regimine) acutorum (Inscr. Περὶ διαίτης ὀξέων, οἱ δὲ περὶ πτισάνης, οἱ δὲ πρὸς τὰς κνιδίας γνώμας).
De morbis popularibus I et III.
De capitis vulneribus.
De officina medici.
De fracturis.
De articulis.
Vectiarius.
Aphorismi.
Lex.
De morbis popularibus II. IV–VII.
De humoribus.
Praesagiorum liber I.
Coa praesagia (fine mutil.).
De arte.
De natura hominis.
De flatibus.
De salubri diaeta (Frgm. Περὶ ἐμέτων. Inc. Ἕξ μῆνας τοὺς χειμερινούς = L. VI 78, 4).
De morbis I.
De affectionibus.
De locis in homine.
De morbo sacro.
De ulceribus.
De haemorroïdibus.
De fistulis.
De victus ratione I–III.
De insomniis.
De morbis II et III.
De natura muliebri.
De septimestri partu.
De octimestri partu.

De genitura.
De natura pueri.
De morbis liber IV.
De mulierum affectibus.
De sterilibus.
De virginum morbis.
De superfoetatione.
De exsectione foetus. De exsectione pueri (I. II).
De anatome.
De dentitione.
De glandulis.
De carnibus.
Praesagiorum liber II.
De alimento.
De corde.
De ossium natura.
De decenti ornatu.
De medico.
Praeceptiones.
De diebus iudicatoriis.
De iudicationibus.
Epistulae (Πρεσβ.).
De febribus (Inc. *wie im* Leydens. Voss. [fol. 10]) (p. 32).
De substantia artis medicae. Definitio artis medicae.

Galenos: (f. 1) *Linguarum sive dictionum exoletarum Hippocratis explicatio* (Sine auctoris nomine. Inscr. Κατὰ στοιχεῖον Ἱπποκράτους λεξικόν. Inc. Ἀγκρομήλη, ἄγκιστρον. Expl. f. 8v ὅτι καὶ ὥρα ἡ φροντὶς ... ἐνιαυτοῦ).
Soranus: (f. 9) *Hippocratis genus et vita secundum Soranum.*
Erotianus, *Vocum Hippocraticarum conlectio.*

München, Hof- und Staatsbibliothek, graec. 72; s. XVI.

(f. 216) *Ad Ptolemaeum regem epistula de hominis fabrica* (Expl. εἰς τὴν κύστιν τὸ ὕδωρ).
(f. 215) *De quattuor elementis et humoribus naturae hominis.*

München, Hof- und Staatsbibliothek, graec. 227; s. XVI.

Damascius: (f. 1) *Expositio in aphorismos Hippocratis. Sectiones VII.*

München, Hof- und Staatsbibliothek, graec. 231; s. XVI.

Galenos, *In Hippocratis epidemiarum libros commentarii I–III* (in Libr. I et II; Inc. mut. μόνον προγνώσεται τὰς γινομένας νόσους = K. XVII A 5, 13. Expl. mut. τῶν ἔνδον τοῦ περιτοναίου μορίων, *also wie im* [Venet.] Marc. App. cl. V 15 [below p. 113], = K. XVII A 791, 19. *Der Codex enthält f.* 1–106^{v} Comm. I–III in Epid. A', f. 106^{v}–228^{v} Comm. I–III in Epid. Γ').

München, Hof- und Staatsbibliothek, graec. 276; s. XII.

(f. 5) **Hippokrates, Galenos**, *Prognostica* (Προγνωστικὸν ἀῤῥώστων συγγραφὲν Ἱππ. καὶ Γαλ. καὶ Πλάτωνος καὶ σοφ. ἰατρῶν).

München, Hof- und Staatsbibliothek, graec. 287; s. XIV, XIV ex., XV.

(f. 153) *De IV aetatibus praenotio.*
(f. 153) *Aphorismi* (Frgm. Ἱππ. πρόγνωσις π. τῶν δ' ὡρῶν = Aph. III 11–14) (III 11–14).

München, Hof- und Staatsbibliothek, graec. 469; s. XIII, XV.
s. XIV (?).
f. 1–50: *nach alter Zählung* φυλλ. ιη'–ϙγ' *am rechten Rande (also vorher die ersten 17 Blätter verloren)*; f. 1–50^{v}: *nach neuerer Zählung am untern Rande, die öfter mehrere Blätter überspringt*; f. 51–55: *nach alter Zählung am rechten Rande* φυλλ. ϙδ'–ϙγ', *nach neuerer am unteren Rande f. 51–55^{v}*; f. 55^{v}: φυλλ. ϙη' *nach alter Zählung am rechten Rande.*

Galenos: (f. 1–50) *In Hippocratis librum de acutorum victu commentarii IV.*

München, Hof- und Staatsbibliothek, graec. 494; s. –.

(f. 14) *De elementis* (Inc. Στοιχεῖα ἀνθρώπου ἴσχοντα ἰσχόμενα ἐνορμῶντα. Expl. γλυκὺ ἁλυκὸν ὀξῶδες καὶ ἄποιον. *Abschrift in Königsberg, Dietz-Nachlaß XVI 31*).

München, Hof- und Staatsbibliothek, graec. 525; ante a. 1336.

(f. 155^{v}–163^{v}) *Aphorismi* (Frgm. ex L. III–VI).

Neapel, Biblioteca Borbonica
Now Napoli, Biblioteca Nazionale Vittorio Emanuele III

Neapel, Biblioteca Borbonica, III C 2 (260); s. –.
= III C 2 (*Census*: 162, nr [0779]).

(f. 1) *De urinis* (Inc. Οὖρον ἄριστόν ἐστιν ὅταν λευκή).

Neapel, Biblioteca Borbonica, 91 (II C 33); s. XV.
Same as **Bibl. di S. Giovanni di Carbonara, 15** below (p. 49).
= II C 32 (*Census*: 162, nr [0782]).

Aphorismi.
Praeceptiones (Frgm.).

Neapel, Biblioteca Borbonica, 187 (II F 30); s. XVI.
Now II F 30 (*Census*: 162, nr [0783]).

(f. 50) *Epistulae* (Πρεσβ.).

Neapel, Biblioteca dei Gerolamini
Now Napoli, Biblioteca statale oratoriana del Monumento nazionale dei Girolamini

Neapel, Bibl. dei Gerolamini, XXII.1; s. XIV, XV.
Now Biblioteca statale oratoriana del Monumento nazionale dei Girolamini, Pil. XXII. nr I (*Census*: 163, nr [0789]).
Same as **Bibl. Oratoriana, 152** below (p. 49).

(f. 133v–135v) *Epistulae* (Epp. 10–13).
(f. 166v–167) *De urinis* (Inc. Ὁκόσοισιν οὖρα παχέα [= Aph. sect. IV nr 69]. Expl. ἀλλ' αὐτῆς καθ' ἑαυτήν).
(f. 161v) *De elementis* (*Wie im* Monac. [494]) (p. 47).

Neapel, Bibliotheca di S. Giovanni di Carbonara

Neapel, Bibl. di S. Giovanni di Carbonara, 15; s. XIV.
Now Biblioteca Nazionale Vittorio Emanuele III, II C 32.
Same as **91 (II C 33)** above (p. 48) (*Census*: 163, nr [0790]).

(f. -) *Excerpta varia.*

Neapel, Bibl. di S. Giovanni di Carbonara, 27; s. XIV.
Now Biblioteca Nazionale Vittorio Emanuele III, III AA 14bis (*Census*: 163, nr [0791]).

Epistulae.

Neapel, Bibliotheca Oratoriana

Neapel, Bibl. Oratoriana, 152; s. XIV, XIV–XV.
Same as **Bibl. dei Gerolamini, XXII.1** above (p. 48) (*Census*: 164, nr [0793]).
Now Biblioteca statale oratoriana del Monumento nazionale dei Girolamini, Pil. XXII. nr I.

De urinis.

Oxford, Bibl. Aedis Christi
Now Oxford, Christ Church Library

Oxford, Bibl. Aedis Christi, 34; s. XI.

(f. 131) *Excerpta varia.*

Oxford, Bibl. Bodleiana

Oxford, Bibl. Bodleiana, Auct. F. Inf. II 3; s. XVIII.
Now MS. Marshall 72 (*Census*: 171, nr [0809]).
See also **Miscell. 132** below (p. 53), and possibly **Auct. T II 3** below.

Aphorismi.
Iusiurandum.
Lex.

Oxford, Bibl. Bodleiana, Auct. T II 3; s. XVIII.
Possibly same as **Auct. F. Inf. II 3** above (*Census*: 171, nr [0810]).
= ? MS. Marshall 72.

Excerpta varia.
Prognosticon (Frgm.).

Oxford, Bibl. Bodleiana, Auct. T II 10; s. XV.
See also **Miscell. 210** below (p. 53).

(f. 82 b) *Epistulae.*

Oxford, Bibl. Bodleiana, Baroccian. 10; s. XV.

(f. 130) *Epistula ad Ptolemaeum regem de sanitate tuenda* (Expl. *wie im* Londin. [Brit. Mus.] Addit. 34060) (p. 34).

Oxford, Bibl. Bodleiana, Baroccian. 51; s. XV.

(f. 61ᵛ) *Epistulae* (Epp. 3. 5–9).

Oxford, Bibl. Bodleiana, Baroccian. 76; s. XV–XVI.

(f. 300–301ᵛ) *Prognosticon* (Frgm. Exc. initii. Expl. πυρετοῦ θάνατον προσημαίνουσι).

Oxford, Bibl. Bodleiana, Baroccian. 88; s. XV–XVI, XV (XVI), XVI.

(f. 47) **Hippokrates, Paulus Italus, Galenos, Athenaeus,** *Prognostica/Excerpta* (Ἱπποκρ. διδασκάλου καὶ Γαλ. σοφοῦ καὶ Παύλου Ἰτάλου καὶ Ἀθηναίου ῥήτορος καὶ Ἰωάννου Τζέτζου διάγνωσις περὶ ἰαλίων [l. ὑαλίων] ἀρρώστων καὶ τελευτῆς ἀνθρώπων. Inc. Τὸ ᾱ ἄσπρον. Expl. σημαίνει καὶ θάνατον).
(f. 47 b) **Hippokrates, Galenos,** *De urinis* (Σύνοψις ἀκριβὴς περὶ οὔρων Ἱππ. καὶ Γαλ. Inc. Ἐὰν ἔστι κλόκιον ἀνθρώπου. Expl. καὶ οὐ σύντομον θάνατον).

Oxford, Bibl. Bodleiana, Baroccian. 131; s. XIV, XIV in.

(f. 477 b) *De pulsibus* (Διάγνωσις ἀκριβὴς τῶν σφυγμῶν. Expl. ταῦτα γάρ εἰσιν Ἱπποκράτους καὶ Γαλ. τῶν ἐπισήμων ἰατρῶν).
(f. 477 b) *Excerpta varia.*
(f. 480) *Excerpta varia.*

Oxford, Bibl. Bodleiana, Baroccian. 150; s. XV, XV in.

(f. 6ᵛ) *Epistula ad Ptolemaeum regem de sanitate tuenda.*

Oxford, Bibl. Bodleiana, Baroccian. 204; s. XV in., XV.

(f. 9) *Iusiurandum* (Iuriiurando se applicat »ἕτερος ὅρκος Ἱπποκράτους«. Inc. αὐτὸν ἐν ἀχράντοισιν. Expl. ὀλβιόδωρον ὑγίειαν. »A corrupt form of the metrical »oath« printed in Kühlew. Hipp. opp. I p. 74«. Scott).
(f. -) *De morbo sacro.*
(f. 9) *Lex.*
(f. 9 b) *De arte.*
(f. 12ᵛ) *De prisca medicina.*
(f. 18) *Praeceptiones.*
(f. 20) *De decenti ornatu.*
(f. 21 b) *De natura hominis.*
(f. 25 b) *De salubri diaeta.*
(f. 27) *De genitura.*
(f. 29) *De natura pueri.*
(f. 36) *De articulis.*
(f. 46) *Epistulae.*
(f. 60 b) *De humoribus.*
(f. 63 b) *De alimento.*
(f. 65) *De ulceribus.*
(f. 74 b) *De morbis I.*
(f. 74 b) *De morbis II et III.*
(f. 74 b) *De morbis liber IV.*
(f. 118) *De affectionibus.*
(f. 126) *De internis affectionibus.*
(f. 144 b) *De victus ratione I–III.*
(f. 165) *De insomniis.*
(f. 167 b) *De visu.*
(f. 168 b) *De diebus iudicatoriis.*
(f. 169 b) *Aphorismi.*
(f. 179) *Prognosticon.*
(f. 185) *De diaeta (regimine) acutorum.*
(f. 199b) *De flatibus.*
(f. 203 b) *Vectiarius.*
(f. 210) *De ossium natura.*
(f. 214) *De fracturis.*
(f. 227) *De officina medici.*
(f. 229) *De exsectione foetus. De exsectione pueri.*
(f. 229 b) *De mulierum affectibus.*
(f. 276) *De sterilibus.*
(f. 284) *De superfoetatione.*

(f. 288 b) *De septimestri partu.*
(f. 290 b) *De octimestri partu.*
(f. 291 b) *De virginum morbis.*
(f. 292) *De natura muliebri.*
(f. 306 b) *De exsectione foetus. De exsectione pueri* (I. II).
(f. 307) *Praesagiorum liber I.*
(f. 307) *Praesagiorum liber II.*
(f. 322) *De fistulis.*
(f. 325) *De haemorroïdibus.*
(f. 326 b) *Coa praesagia.*
(f. 333ᵛ) *De morbis popularibus I et III.*
(f. 333ᵛ) *De morbis popularibus II. IV–VII.*

Galenos: (f. 1) *Linguarum sive dictionum exoletarum Hippocratis explicatio* (»Consentit plerumque, sed paulo contractius cum Galeni lexico«).
Theophilus: (f. 1) *Commentarius in Hippocratis aphorismos* (Initium solum).
Soranus: (f. 8) *Hippocratis genus et vita secundum Soranum.*
Erotianus, *Vocum Hippocraticarum conlectio.*

Oxford, Bibl. Bodleiana, Baroccian. 224; s. XV in., XV.

(f. 3) *De mensibus* (Inc. Πρῶτον μὲν περὶ τῆς ἐγκυκλίου σφαίρας. Expl. περὶ μηνῶν καὶ ὀνήσιμος ἄγαν).

Oxford, Bibl. Bodleiana, Canonician. 1; s. XVI.

(f. 66) *Ad Ptolemaeum regem epistula de hominis fabrica* (Inc. Οὗτος οὖν ὁ κόσμος συνίσταται ἐκ τεσσ. στοιχ.).
(f. 119 b) *Hippocratis Ad Galenum discipulum liber de pulsibus et de temperamentis corporis humani* (Inscr. Περὶ τοῦ σώματος τοῦ ἀνθρώπου πῶς συνίσταται. Inc. Τὸ σῶμα τοῦ ἀνθρώπου συνίσταται ἐκ τεσσάρων στοιχείων. Expl. εἰς τὴν ἀναλυτικὴν ἐνέργεια τῶν βρωμάτων τῶν ἐν αὐτῷ).

Oxford, Bibl. Bodleiana, Clarkian. 16 (18378); s. XIV.
= MS. E. D. Clarke 16 (*Census*: 175, nr [0835]).

(f. 88 b) *Epistula ad Ptolemaeum regem de sanitate tuenda.*

Oxford, Bibl. Bodleiana, Ger. Langbainii Advers. 2; s. –.
Now MS. Langbaine 2 (*Census*: 175, nr [0836]).

(f. 69 b) *Epistula ad Ptolemaeum regem de sanitate tuenda* (Expl. mut. πόνοις καὶ καμάτοις καὶ ἀφροδισίοις).

Oxford, Bibl. Bodleiana, Miscell. 130; s. XVII.
Now MS. Auct. F. inf. 2. 1 (*Census*: 178, nr [0853]).

(f. 315) *De insomniis.*

Oxford, Bibl. Bodleiana, Miscell. 132; s. XVI.
Same as **Auct. F. Inf. II 3** above (p. 49), and possibly also **Auct. T II 3** above (p. 50).
Now MS. Marshall 72 (*Census*: 178, nr [0854]).

(f. 1) *Iusiurandum.*
(f. 2 b) *Lex.*
(f. 4 b) *Aphorismi.*
(f. 58 b) *Prognosticon.*

Oxford, Bibl. Bodleiana, Miscell. 210; s. –.
Same as **Auct T II 10** above (p. 50) (*Census*: 178, nr [0857]).
= MS. Auct. T. 2. 10.

Epistulae.

Oxford, Bibl. Bodleiana, d'Orvillian. X 1. 1. 3; s. XV ex.
Now MS. D'Orville 3 (*Census*: 179, nr [0865]).
See [**Amsterdam, Universitäts-Bibliothek, Amstelodam.** ?] above (p. 5).

Galenos: (f. 144) *Linguarum sive dictionum exoletarum Hippocratis explicatio.*
Erotianus: (f. 166) *Vocum Hippocraticarum conlectio.*

Oxford, Bibl. Bodleiana, Orvillian. X 1. 4. 29; s. XVIII in.
Now MS. D'Orville 131 (*Census*: 179, nr [0867]).

De remediis.

Oxford, Bibl. Bodleiana, Roe 14 (260); s. XV.
See **Roe 14 (Bodl. 260)** below.
= MS. Roe 14 (*Census*: 180, nr [0870]).

(f. 52) *Sententiae de vita et morte* (Inc. *und* Expl. *wie im* Lond. Medical Society [HH i 21. 22 = We 28. 29]) (p. 35).

Oxford, Bibl. Bodleiana, Roe 14 (Bodl. 260); s. XV.
Same as **Roe 14 (260)** above.
= MS. Roe 14 (*Census*: 180, nr [0871]).

Theophilus: (f. 87ᵛ) *Commentarius in Hippocratis aphorismos* (= Dtz. II 245–543 ἴαμα).

Oxford, Bibl. Bodleiana, Roe XIV (260); s. XV.
Same as **Roe 14 (260)** above.
= MS. Roe 14 (*Census*: 180, nr [0874]).

(f. 73) *De decenti ornatu* (Frgm. Inc. Χρὴ τὸν ἰατρόν = L. IX 236, 3).
(f. 87ᵛ) *Aphorismi*.

Padua, Bibl. Canonicor. Lateranens.

[Padua, Bibl. Canonicor. Lateranens.].
Now Oxford, Bodleian Library, Holkham Gr. 92 (*Census*: 187–188, nr [0886]).
Same as **Holkham 282** above (p. 26) and **[Padua, Bibl. S. Joannis in Viridario plut. XVII]** below.

De genitura.

Padua, Bibl. S. Joannis in Viridario

Padua, Bibl. S. Joannis in Viridario, ad dextr. plut. XVII.
Verbleib unbekannt. Holkham nr. 282 *nach Zuschrift von* Emil Jacobs (*Zu vgl.* R. Foerster, Philologus 42, 162).
Same as **Holkham 282** (p. 26), and **[Padua, Bibl. Canonicor. Lateranens.]** above.
Now Oxford, Bodleian Library, Holkham Gr. 92 (*Census* 193–194, nr [0903]).

Aphorismi.
De genitura.
De natura hominis.
De virginum morbis.
Opera varia.
Prognosticon.

Palermo, Biblioteca nazionale
Now Palermo, Biblioteca centrale della Regione siciliana «Alberto Bombace»

Palermo, Biblioteca nazionale, XIII C 3; s. –, XVI.

(f. 1–44ᵛ) **Hippokrates**, **Galenos**, *Jatrosophium* (Ἰατροσόφ. Ἱππ. καὶ Γαλ. καὶ ἑτέρων φιλοσόφων καὶ ἰατρῶν. Inc. Περὶ ἤθους ἰατρῶν. Ποδαπὸν δεῖ εἶναι τὸν ἰητρόν. Expl. ἐν οὔρῳ, ἐν πτύσμασιν, ἐν ἱδρῶτι).
(f. 49–55) *Aphorismi* (c. comm.).
(f. 121–238) **Hippokrates**, **Galenos**, *Jatrosophium/Iatrosophia* (Inscr. Ἀνθολόγιον ἰατροσοφικὸν τοῦ Ἱππ. τοῦ Κῴου καὶ Γαλ. ... καὶ ἑτέρ. ἰατρῶν).

Paris, Bibl. regia

[Paris, B. R. 120 ap. Montf. II 902].
= Paris, Bibliothèque nationale de France, *Coislinianus* 163 below (p. 56) (*Census*: 195, nr [0909]).

Galenos, *In Hippocratis de humoribus librum commentarii III.*

Paris, Bibl. de Paris

Paris, Bibl. de Paris, 4; s. XVI.
= Paris, Bibliothèque Mazarine, 4454 (*Census*: 197–198, nr [0913]).

(f. 159ᵛ) *Epistulae.*

Paris, Bibl. Facult. Méd. / Bibl. Facult. Medic./ Faculté de Méd.
Now Paris, Bibliothèque Interuniversitaire de Santé-BIU Santé.

Paris, Bibl. Facult. Med., 14; s. XVII.
Same as **Bibl. Facult Medic. 14** below.
= MS 44 (*Census*: 199, nr [0920]).

Lexicon Hippocratis.

Paris, Bibl. Facult. Medic. 14; s. XVII.
= MS 44 (*Census*: 199, nr [0920]).
See also **Paris, Bibl. Facult. Med., 14** above, and possibly also **Faculté de Méd.** below.

Galenos: (f. 73) *In Hippocratis de humoribus librum commentarii III* (e cod. Coisl. 163 descr.).

Paris, Faculté de Méd.
Possibly same as **Bibl. Facult Medic. 14** above.
= ? MS 44 (*Census*: 198, nr [0916]).

Apollonius Citiensis, *Commentarius in Hippocratis de articulis, libri III* (*vgl.* Dietz, Schol. in Hipp. et Gal. I prf. p. XI): II.15.

Paris, Bibl. Nationale, Coislin.
Now Paris, Bibliothèque nationale de France, Coisliniani

Paris, Bibl. Nationale, Coislin., 163; a. 1560.
See also **[Paris, B. R. 120 ap. Montf. II 902]** above (p. 55).

Galenos: (f. 73) *In Hippocratis de humoribus librum commentarii III.*

Paris, Bibl. Nationale, Coislin., 321; s. XVI.
See also **[321 (?)]** below.

(f. 115) *Hippocratis ad Ptolemaeum epistula.*

[Paris, Bibl. Nationale, Coislin., 321 (?)].
Same as **Coislin 321** above (*Census*: 205, nr [0946]).

Epistula ad Ptolemaeum regem de sanitate tuenda.

Paris, Bibl. Nationale, Coislin., 335; s. XV.
See possibly **[335]** below.

(f. 21–60) **Galenos,** *Iatrosophia* (Jatros. Gal. Hipp. Melet. Cap. DCIV).
(f. 75) **Galenos, Hippokrates, Meletius monachus**, *Iatrosophia/Excerpta varia* (Jatros. Gal. Hipp. et Melet. Cap. DCIV.

[Paris, Bibl. Nationale, Coislin., 335].
= ? **Coislin 335** above (*Census*: 205–206, nr [0951]).

De genitura.

Paris, Bibl. Nationale, Parisin.
Now Paris, Bibliothèque nationale de France, *graeci*

Paris, Bibl. Nationale, Parisin. 36; s. XIV–XV.
See also **[3170 (?)]** below (p. 88).

(f. 17) *Prognosticon.*
(f. 30) *Aphorismi.*
(f. 55) *De victus ratione I–III.*
(f. 95) *De venae sectione* (Inc. Ἐν πάσῃ ἡμέρᾳ).

Paris, Bibl. Nationale, Parisin. 396; s. XIII.

(f. 460) *Prognosticon* (prooem.).
(f. 707) *De septimanis* (Frgm. Inc. *und* Expl. *wie im* Berol. Phillipps. 1529 [above p. 11]).

Paris, Bibl. Nationale, Parisin. 985; s. XV, XVI.

(f. 302) *Hippocratis et Galeni philosophia De natura hominis* (Λέξεις Ἱππ. πρὸς Γαλ. τὸν ἑαυτοῦ μαθητὴν περὶ ἀνθρώπου. Περὶ διαπλάσεως ἀνθρώπου).

Paris, Bibl. Nationale, Parisin. 1297; s. XVI.

(f. 63) *Aphorismi.*

Paris, Bibl. Nationale, Parisin. 1327; a. 1562.

(f. 208v) *Epistulae* (Epistulae ad Damaget.).

[Paris, Bibl. Nationale, Parisin. 1444 (?)].
= ? **2140–2146** below (pp. 60–70) and **2255** below (p. 78) (*Census*: 210–211, nr [0996]).

De articulis.

Paris, Bibl. Nationale, Parisin. 1630; s. XIV.

(f. 146) *Epistula ad Ptolemaeum regem de sanitate tuenda.*
(f. 202[v]) *Ad Ptolemaeum regem epistula de hominis fabrica.*

[Paris, Bibl. Nationale, Parisin. 1667 (?)].
= ? **1884** below (p. 59) (*Census*: 211, nr [1002]).

De febribus.

Paris, Bibl. Nationale, Parisin. 1760; s. XV.

(f. 146, f. 205) *Epistulae* (Artax. et Hipp. epp.).

[Paris, Bibl. Nationale, Parisin. 1848 ?].
= ? **1884** below (p. 59) (*Census*: 212, nr [1010]).

Aphorismi.

Paris, Bibl. Nationale, Parisin. 1849; s. XIV.

(f. 111) *De articulis* (c. comm. Gal.).
(f. 147[v]) *De fracturis* (c. comm. Gal.).
(f. 175[v]) *De officina medici* (c. comm. Gal.).

Galenos:
(f. 111) *In Hippocratis de articulis librum commentarii IV.*
(f. 147[v]) *In Hippocratis librum de fracturis commentarii III.*
(f. 175[v]) *In Hippocratis librum de officina medici commentarii III.*

Paris, Bibl. Nationale, Parisin. 1868; s. XIV, XV.

De salubri diaeta (Frgm. Inc. Ὁκόσους δὲ δίψαι = L. VI 84, 15).
(f. 368) *De genitura.*
(f. 368) *De natura hominis* (Frgm.).
(f. 369[v]) *De natura pueri.*
(f. 375[v]–376[v]) *De articulis* (cf. L. IV 76).
(f. 377) *Lex.*
(f. 377) *De arte.*
(f. 379[v]–381) *De prisca medicina* (Frgm.).
(f. 382. 391) *De articulis* (cf. L. IV 76).
(f. 397) *De prisca medicina* (Frgm. imperf. L. IV 76).

Erotianus, *Vocum Hippocraticarum conlectio.*

Paris, Bibl. Nationale, Parisin. 1883; s. XIV.

(f. 35ᵛ) *De elementis.*
(f. 66ᵛ) *Prognosticon* (»Libri III«).
(f. 74ᵛ) *Aphorismi* (c. comm. Theophil.; init. mutil.).

Theophilus: (f. 74ᵛ–156) *Commentarius in Hippocratis aphorismos* (Sine auctor. nomine. Inc. mutil. Τεχνικῆς φάμεν. *Vgl.* Costomiris, Rev. des ét. gr. II [1889] p. 357).

Paris, Bibl. Nationale, Parisin. 1884; a. 1503.
See also (possibly) **[1667 (?)]** and **[1848 ?]** (p. 58) above, and **[1884]**, **[1884 (?)]**, **[1885]**, **[1885 (?)]** below.

(f. 78ᵛ) *Prognosticon.*
(f. 92ᵛ) *De febribus* (Inc. Τοῦτό σοι τὸ τρίτον ἐπίταγμα).
(f. 158) *Aphorismi* (c. comm. Gal.).

Galenos: (f. 158) *Hippocratis aphorismi et Galeni in eos commentarii VII.*

[Paris, Bibl. Nationale, Parisin. 1884; a. 1403].
Same as **1884** above (*Census*: 213, nr [1016]).

(f. 95) *Epistulae.*

[Paris, Bibl. Nationale, Parisin. 1884 (?)].
Same as **1884** above (*Census*: 213, nr [1017]).

Epistula ad Ptolemaeum regem de sanitate tuenda.

[Paris, Bibl. Nationale, Parisin. 1885; s. XVI].
Possibly same as **1884** above (*Census*: 213, nr [1018]).

(f. 35ᵛ) *Epistulae.*

[Paris, Bibl. Nationale, Parisin. 1885 (?)].
Possibly same as **1884** above (*Census*: 213, nr [1019]).

De febribus.

Paris, Bibl. Nationale, Parisin. 1995; s. XV.

(f. 190) *Hippiatricorum libri XVI* (Sostrati et Hippocratis collectanea hippiatr.).

[Paris, Bibl. Nationale, Parisin. 2030; s. XVI ?].
Same as **2330** below (p. 83) (*Census*: 214, nr [1027]).

Praesagiorum liber I.
Praesagiorum liber II.

Paris, Bibl. Nationale, Parisin. 2047; s. XV.

(f. 13^v) *Ad Ptolemaeum regem epistula de hominis fabrica.*
(f. 16) *Iusiurandum.*

Paris, Bibl. Nationale, Parisin. 2091; s. XV.

(f. 118) *Hippiatricorum libri XVI* (Hippiatr. ex Onosandro et Hippocrate).

Paris, Bibl. Nationale, Parisin. 2140; s. XII–XIII.
Possibly same as **[1444 (?)]** above (p. 57). See also **[2140]**, and possibly **[2146 (?]** (p. 70) below.

(f. 9^v) *Iusiurandum.*
(f. 9^v) *Lex.*
(f. 10^v) *De arte.*
(f. 13) *De prisca medicina.*
(f. 19) *Praeceptiones.*
(f. 20^v) *De decenti ornatu.*
(f. 22^v) *De natura hominis.*
(f. 28) *De genitura.*
(f. 30) *De natura pueri.*
(f. 38) *De articulis.*
(f. 62^v) *De humoribus.*
(f. 62^v) *De alimento.*
(f. 66^v) *De ulceribus.*
(f. 70^v) *De morbo sacro.*
(f. 75^v) *De morbis liber IV.*
(f. 75^v) *De morbis I.*
(f. 75^v) *De morbis II et III.*
(f. 117) *De affectionibus.*
(f. 126) *De internis affectionibus.*
(f. 146) *De victus ratione I–III.*

(f. 169) *De insomniis.*
(f. 171^{v}) *De visu.*
(f. 172^{v}) *De diebus iudicatoriis.*
(f. 174) *Aphorismi.*
(f. 184) *Prognosticon.*
(f. 190^{v}) *De diaeta (regimine) acutorum.*
(f. 206) *De flatibus.*
(f. 209^{v}) *Vectiarius.*
(f. 216) *De ossium natura.*
(f. 220) *De fracturis.*
(f. 234) *De officina medici.*
(f. 237^{v}) *De mulierum affectibus.*
(f. 237) *De exsectione foetus. De exsectione pueri* (I).
(f. 291^{v}) *De sterilibus.*
(f. 300) *De superfoetatione.*
(f. 304) *De septimestri partu.*
(f. 306) *De octimestri partu.*
(f. 307) *De virginum morbis.*
(f. 308) *De natura muliebri.*
(f. 323^{v}) *De exsectione foetus. De exsectione pueri* (II).
(f. 324^{v}) *Praesagiorum liber I.*
(f. 338^{v}) *De fistulis.*
(f. 340^{v}) *De haemorroïdibus.*
(f. 342^{v}) *Coa praesagia.*
(f. 349) *De morbis popularibus II. IV–VII.*
(f. 349) *De morbis popularibus I et III.*
(f. 324^{v}) *Praesagiorum liber II.*
(f. 414) *Epistulae.*

Galenos: (f. 1) *Linguarum sive dictionum exoletarum Hippocratis explicatio.*
Soranus: (f. 8^{v}) *Hippocratis genus et vita secundum Soranum.*

[Paris, Bibl. Nationale, Parisin. 2140].
Same as **2140** above (*Census*: 216, nr [1042]).

(f. -) *De salubri diaeta.*

Paris, Bibl. Nationale, Parisin. 2141; s. XV.
Possibly same as **[1444 (?)]** above (p. 57). See also **[2141]** (p. 63) below.

(f. 8^{v}) *Iusiurandum.*
(f. 8^{v}) *Lex.*

(f. 9v) *De arte.*
(f. 11v) *De prisca medicina.*
(f. 16v) *Praeceptiones.*
(f. 18) *De decenti ornatu.*
(f. 20) *De natura hominis.*
(f. 25v) *De genitura.*
(f. 27v) *De natura pueri.*
(f. 35) *De articulis.*
(f. 57v) *De humoribus.*
(f. 60v) *De alimento.*
(f. 62) *De ulceribus.*
(f. 65v) *De morbo sacro.*
(f. 70v) *De morbis I.*
(f. 70v) *De morbis II et III.*
(f. 70v) *De morbis liber IV.*
(f. 109) *De affectionibus.*
(f. 117v) *De internis affectionibus.*
(f. 136) *De victus ratione I–III.*
(f. 155) *De insomniis.*
(f. 157v) *De visu.*
(f. 158) *De diebus iudicatoriis.*
(f. 159v) *Aphorismi.*
(f. 167) *Prognosticon.*
(f. 172) *De diaeta (regimine) acutorum.*
(f. 184) *De flatibus.*
(f. 186v) *Vectiarius.*
(f. 191v) *De ossium natura.*
(f. 195) *De fracturis.*
(f. 205) *De officina medici.*
(f. 207v) *De mulierum affectibus.*
(f. 207) *De exsectione foetus. De exsectione pueri* (I).
(f. 248) *De sterilibus.*
(f. 254) *De superfoetatione.*
(f. 257v) *De septimestri partu.*
(f. 259) *De octimestri partu.*
(f. 260v) *De natura muliebri.*
(f. 260) *De virginum morbis.*
(f. 273v) *De exsectione foetus. De exsectione pueri* (II).
(f. 274) *Praesagiorum liber I.*
(f. 274) *Praesagiorum liber II.*
(f. 285v) *De fistulis.*

(f. 287v) *De haemorroïdibus.*
(f. 288v) *Coa praesagia.*
(f. 293v) *De morbis popularibus I et III.*
(f. 293v) *De morbis popularibus II. IV–VII.*
(f. 339) *Epistulae.*

Galenos: (f. 1) *Linguarum sive dictionum exoletarum Hippocratis explicatio.*
Soranus: (f. 8) *Hippocratis genus et vita secundum Soranum.*
Erotianus, *Vocum Hippocraticarum conlectio.*

[Paris, Bibl. Nationale, Parisin. 2141; s. XV].
Same as **2141** above (*Census*: 216, nr [1044]).

(f. -) *De salubri diaeta.*

Paris, Bibl. Nationale, Parisin. 2142; s. XIII–XIV.
Possibly same as **[1444 (?)]** above (p. 57). See also **[2142]** (p. 64) and **[2242 (?)]** (p. 75).

Coa praesagia.
De humoribus.
(f. 12v) *Iusiurandum.*
(f. 13) *Lex.*
(f. 13v) *De arte.*
(f. 17) *De prisca medicina.*
(f. 25v) *De decenti ornatu.*
(f. 28) *De natura hominis.*
(f. 36) *De natura pueri.*
(f. 44v) *De genitura.*
(f. 44v) *De articulis.*
(f. 82) *Vectiarius.*
(f. 86v) *De alimento.*
(f. 89v) *De ulceribus.*
(f. 97) *De morbo sacro.*
(f. 107v) *De morbis I.*
(f. 107v) *De morbis II et III.*
(f. 107v) *De morbis liber IV.*
(f. 198v) *De internis affectionibus.*
(f. 231v) *De victus ratione I–III.*
(f. 268v) *De insomniis.*
(f. 272v) *De visu.*
(f. 274v) *De diebus iudicatoriis.*

(f. 277) *Aphorismi.*
(f. 292^{v}) *Prognosticon.*
(f. 302^{v}) *De diaeta (regimine) acutorum.*
(f. 319) *De flatibus.*
(f. 322) *Vectiarius.*
(f. 328^{v}) *De ossium natura.*
(f. 333) *De fracturis.*
(f. 347^{v}) *De officina medici.*
(f. 351) *De mulierum affectibus.*
(f. 406^{v}) *De sterilibus.*
(f. 415^{v}) *De superfoetatione.*
(f. 420) *De septimestri partu.*
(f. 422^{v}) *De octimestri partu.*
(f. 423^{v}) *De virginum morbis.*
(f. 424) *De natura muliebri.*
(f. 441) *De exsectione foetus. De exsectione pueri* (I).
(f. 442) *Praesagiorum liber I.*
(f. 442) *Praesagiorum liber II.*
(f. 456) *De fistulis.*
(f. 458) *De haemorroïdibus.*
(f. 466) *De morbis popularibus I et III.*
(f. 466) *De morbis popularibus II. IV–VII.*
(f. 530) *Epistulae.*
(f. 547^{v}) *De septimanis* (Frgm. Inc. ... οὐκ ἔχει ἑπτὰ μέρεα. Expl. ἀνὴρ πρεσβύτης γέρων; cf. L. IX 433 s.).

Galenos: (f. 1) *Linguarum sive dictionum exoletarum Hippocratis explicatio.*
Soranus: (f. 12) *Hippocratis genus et vita secundum Soranum.*
Erotianus, *Vocum Hippocraticarum conlectio.*

[Paris, Bibl. Nationale, Parisin. 2142; s. XIII–XIV].
Same as **2142** above (*Census*: 217, nr [1046]).

(f. -) *De salubri diaeta.*
(f. 350) *De exsectione foetus. De exsectione pueri* (II).

Paris, Bibl. Nationale, Parisin. 2143; s. XIV.
Possibly same as **[1444 (?)]** above (p. 57). See also **[2143]** and **[2143 (?)]** below (p. 66), possibly in addition to **[2148]** below (p. 71).

De natura hominis.
(f. 11) *Iusiurandum.*

(f. 11^{v}) *Lex.*
(f. 15^{v}) *De prisca medicina.*
(f. 21^{v}) *Praeceptiones.*
(f. 23) *De decenti ornatu.*
(f. 31) *De genitura.*
(f. 33^{v}) *De natura pueri.*
(f. 39^{v}) *De articulis.*
(f. 62) *De humoribus.*
(f. 65^{v}) *De alimento.*
(f. 67) *De ulceribus.*
(f. 71^{v}) *De morbo sacro.*
(f. 76^{v}) *De morbis I.*
(f. 76^{v}) *De morbis II et III.*
(f. 76^{v}) *De morbis liber IV.*
(f. 111^{v}) *De affectionibus.*
(f. 118^{v}) *De internis affectionibus.*
(f. 136) *De victus ratione I–III.*
(f. 155^{v}) *De insomniis.*
(f. 158) *De visu.*
(f. 159) *De diebus iudicatoriis.*
(f. 160^{v}) *Aphorismi.*
(f. 169) *Prognosticon.*
(f. 175^{v}) *De diaeta (regimine) acutorum.*
(f. 192) *De flatibus.*
(f. 195^{v}) *Vectiarius.*
(f. 201^{v}) *De ossium natura.*
(f. 205^{v}) *De fracturis.*
(f. 219) *De officina medici.*
(f. 221^{v}) *De exsectione foetus. De exsectione pueri* (I. II).
(f. 222) *De mulierum affectibus.*
(f. 267) *De sterilibus.*
(f. 275) *De superfoetatione.*
(f. 278^{v}) *De septimestri partu.*
(f. 280^{v}) *De octimestri partu.*
(f. 281^{v}) *De virginum morbis.*
(f. 282) *De natura muliebri.*
(f. 298) *De exsectione foetus. De exsectione pueri* (I. II).
(f. 298^{v}) *Praesagiorum liber I.*
(f. 298^{v}) *Praesagiorum liber II.*
(f. 311^{v}) *De fistulis.*
(f. 314) *De haemorroïdibus.*

(f. 315) *Coa praesagia.*
(f. 321) *De morbis popularibus I et III.*
(f. 321) *De morbis popularibus II. IV–VII.*
(f. 375) *Epistulae.*

Galenos: (f. 1v) *Linguarum sive dictionum exoletarum Hippocratis explicatio.*
Soranus: (f. 10) *Hippocratis genus et vita secundum Soranum.*
Erotianus, *Vocum Hippocraticarum conlectio.*

[Paris, Bibl. Nationale, Parisin. 2143; s. XIV].
Same as **2143** above (*Census*: 218, nr [1049]).

(f. -) *De salubri diaeta.*

[Paris, Bibl. Nationale, Parisin. 2143 (?); s. XIV].
Same as **2143** above (*Census*: 218, nr [1050]).

De arte.

Paris, Bibl. Nationale, Parisin. 2144; s. XIV.
Possibly same as **[1444 (?)]** above (p. 57). See also **[2144]** below, and possibly **[2154]** below (p. 72).

(f. 13) *Iusiurandum.*
(f. 13) *Lex.*
(f. 14) *De arte.*
(f. 17) *De prisca medicina.*
(f. 25) *Praeceptiones.*
(f. 27) *De decenti ornatu.*
(f. 29) *De natura hominis.*
(f. 34v) *De genitura.*
(f. 36v) *De natura pueri.*
(f. 44v) *De articulis.*
(f. 71) *De humoribus.*
(f. 74) *De alimento.*
(f. 75v) *De ulceribus.*
(f. 80) *De morbo sacro.*
(f. 85) *De morbis I.*
(f. 85) *De morbis liber IV.*
(f. 85v) *De morbis II et III.*
(f. 127v) *De affectionibus.*
(f. 138v) *De internis affectionibus.*

(f. 158ᵛ) *De victus ratione I–III.*
(f. 183ᵛ) *De insomniis.*
(f. 186ᵛ) *De visu.*
(f. 187ᵛ) *De diebus iudicatoriis.*
(f. 188) *Aphorismi.*
(f. 208) *Prognosticon.*
(f. 215) *De diaeta (regimine) acutorum.*
(f. 228) *De flatibus.*
(f. 231) *Vectiarius.*
(f. 236) *De ossium natura.*
(f. 240) *De fracturis.*
(f. 250ᵛ) *De officina medici.*
(f. 252ᵛ) *De exsectione foetus. De exsectione pueri* (I).
(f. 253) *De mulierum affectibus.*
(f. 295) *De sterilibus.*
(f. 302) *De superfoetatione.*
(f. 306) *De septimestri partu.*
(f. 308) *De octimestri partu.*
(f. 309ᵛ) *De natura muliebri.*
(f. 309) *De virginum morbis.*
(f. 323) *De exsectione foetus. De exsectione pueri* (II).
(f. 323ᵛ) *Praesagiorum liber I.*
(f. 323ᵛ) *Praesagiorum liber II.*
(f. 337) *De haemorroïdibus.*
(f. 335ᵛ) *De fistulis.*
(f. 338) *Coa praesagia.*
(f. 343ᵛ) *De morbis popularibus I et III.*
(f. 343ᵛ) *De morbis popularibus II. IV–VII.*
(f. 390) *Epistulae.*

Galenos: (f. 1) *Linguarum sive dictionum exoletarum Hippocratis explicatio.*
Soranus: (f. 12) *Hippocratis genus et vita secundum Soranum.*
Erotianus, *Vocum Hippocraticarum conlectio.*

[Paris, Bibl. Nationale, Parisin. 2144; s. XIV].
Same as **2144** above (*Census*: 219, nr [1052]).

(f. -) *De salubri diaeta.*

Paris, Bibl. Nationale, Parisin. 2145; s. XV.
Possibly same as **[1444 (?)]** above (p. 57). See also **[2145]** (p. 69), **[2154]** (possibly, p. 72), **2545 (? = 2145** ? **cf. Kühn l. 1)**, **[2545 (?) = 2145** ?] and **[2545 (? = 2145** ?)] below (all p. 85).

(f. 14) *Iusiurandum.*
(f. 14ᵛ) *Lex.*
(f. 15) *De arte.*
(f. 19ᵛ) *De prisca medicina.*
(f. 28ᵛ) *Praeceptiones.*
(f. 31) *De decenti ornatu.*
(f. 43) *De genitura.*
(f. 46ᵛ) *De natura pueri.*
(f. 58) *De articulis.*
(f. 96ᵛ) *De humoribus.*
(f. 100) *De alimento.*
(f. 102ᵛ) *De ulceribus.*
(f. 108ᵛ) *De morbo sacro.*
(f. 116ᵛ) *De morbis I.*
(f. 116ᵛ) *De morbis liber IV.*
(f. 116ᵛ) *De morbis II et III.*
(f. 175) *De affectionibus.*
(f. 188ᵛ) *De internis affectionibus.*
(f. 217) *De victus ratione I–III.*
(f. 247ᵛ) *De insomniis.*
(f. 251ᵛ) *De visu.*
(f. 253) *De diebus iudicatoriis.*
(f. 255) *Aphorismi.*
(f. 268ᵛ) *Prognosticon.*
(f. 277ᵛ) *De diaeta (regimine) acutorum.*
(f. 298) *De flatibus.*
(f. 303) *Vectiarius.*
(f. 312) *De ossium natura.*
(f. 317ᵛ) *De fracturis.*
(f. 336ᵛ) *De officina medici.*
(f. 340) *De exsectione foetus. De exsectione pueri* (I).
(f. 341) *De mulierum affectibus.*
(f. 409) *De sterilibus.*
(f. 420ᵛ) *De superfoetatione.*
(f. 426ᵛ) *De septimestri partu.*
(f. 429) *De octimestri partu.*

(f. 430v) *De virginum morbis.*
(f. 431v) *De natura muliebri.*
(f. 452v) *De exsectione foetus. De exsectione pueri* (II).
(f. 453v) *Praesagiorum liber I.*
(f. 453v) *Praesagiorum liber II.*
(f. 473) *De fistulis.*
(f. 476) *De haemorroïdibus.*
(f. 477v) *Coa praesagia.*
(f. 487) *De morbis popularibus I et III.*
(f. 487) *De morbis popularibus II. IV–VII.*
(f. 573) *Epistulae.*

Galenos: (f. 1) *Linguarum sive dictionum exoletarum Hippocratis explicatio.*
Soranus, *Hippocratis genus et vita secundum Soranum.*
Erotianus, *Vocum Hippocraticarum conlectio.*

[Paris, Bibl. Nationale, Parisin. 2145; s. XV].
Same as **2145** above (*Census*: 218, nr [1054]).

(f. -) *De salubri diaeta.*

Paris, Bibl. Nationale, Parisin. 2146; s. XVI.
Possibly same as **[1444 (?)]** above (p. 57). See also **[2146]**, **[2146 (?)]** (p. 70) and below **[2546 (? = 2146 ?)]** (p. 86).

De capitis vulneribus.
(f. 1) *Iusiurandum.*
(f. 1v) *Lex.*
(f. 2) *Aphorismi.*
(f. 14v) *Prognosticon.*
(f. 22) *De diaeta (regimine) acutorum.*
(f. 41v) *De officina medici.*
(f. 44v) *De fracturis.*
(f. 61) *De articulis.*
(f. 103v) *De aëre, aquis et locis.*
(f. 110) *De morbis popularibus I et III.*
(f. 110) *De morbis popularibus II. IV–VII.*
(f. 179v) *De natura hominis.*
(f. 187) *De natura pueri.*
(f. 198v) *De genitura.*
(f. 201v) *De superfoetatione.*
(f. 206v) *De septimestri partu.*

(f. 207ᵛ) *De octimestri partu.*
(f. 210ᵛ) *De virginum morbis.*
(f. 211) *De natura muliebri.*
(f. 227ᵛ) *De dentitione.*
(f. 228ᵛ) *Ad Ptolemaeum regem epistula de hominis fabrica* (»de partibus corporis humani«).
(f. 241ᵛ) *De mulierum affectibus.*
(f. 318) *De exsectione foetus. De exsectione pueri* (II).
(f. 318ᵛ) *De medico.*
(f. 321) *De diebus decretoriis.*
(f. 324ᵛ) *De corde.*
(f. 326) *De carnibus.*
(f. 331) *De glandulis.*
(f. 333ᵛ) *De anatome.*
(f. 334) *Epistulae.*

[Paris, Bibl. Nationale, Parisin. 2146; s. XVI].
Same as **2146** above (*Census*: 218–219, nr [1056]).

(f. -) *De salubri diaeta.*
(f. 307ᵛ) *De sterilibus.*

[Paris, Bibl. Nationale, Parisin. 2146 (?); s. XVI].
Same as **2146** above, and possibly **2140** above (p. 60) (*Census*: 219, nr [1057]).

De locis in homine (= 2146).
De visu (= ? 2140).
De iudicationibus (= ? 2146 [= ? *De diebus iudicatoriis*]).

Paris, Bibl. Nationale, Parisin. 2147; s. XVI.
See also **[2147]** and **[2147 (?)]** below.

Aphorismi (Frgm. ἐξήγησις Στεφάνου. Inc. ἐπὶ περιπνευμονίῃ φρενῖτις).
(f. 1) *De natura pueri* (imperf.).
(f. 6) *De natura hominis* (Expl. Σχεδὸν δὲ καὶ πάντα).

[Paris, Bibl. Nationale, Parisin. 2147; s. XVI].
Same as **2147** above (*Census*: 219, nr [1059]).

(f. -) *De salubri diaeta.*

[Paris, Bibl. Nationale, Parisin. 2147 (?); s. XVI].
Same as **2147** above (*Census*: 219, nr [1060]).

De genitura.

Paris, Bibl. Nationale, Parisin. 2148; s. XV.

(f. 1) *Iusiurandum.*
(f. 1) *Lex.*
(f. 1) *De arte.*
(f. 7) *De morbis I.*
(f. 7) *De morbis II et III.*
(f. 7) *De morbis liber IV.*
(f. 26ᵛ) *De affectionibus.*
(f. 30ᵛ) *De internis affectionibus.*
(f. 39) *De victus ratione I–III.*
(f. 50) *De diaeta (regimine) acutorum.*
(f. 56ᵛ) *De fistulis.*
(f. 57ᵛ) *De ulceribus.*
(f. 59) *De unguentis.*
(f. 61ᵛ) *Praesagiorum liber II* (Frgm. Inc. ὅσοι μὲν ἢ γέροντες = L. IX 26, 16).

Erotianus, *Vocum Hippocraticarum conlectio.*

[Paris, Bibl. Nationale, Parisin. 2148; ns. XV, XVI].
Possibly same as **2143** above (p. 64) (*Census*: 220, nr [1062]).

Aphorismi.
(f. 48) *De insomniis.*
(f. 49ᵛ) *De visu.*
(f. 50) *De diebus iudicatoriis.*
(f. 57) *De haemorroïdibus.*
(f. 59ᵛ) *De morbo sacro.*

Paris, Bibl. Nationale, Parisin. 2149; s. XVI.
See also **2149 (?)** below.

(f. 1) *Aphorismi* (c. comm. Theophili).
(f. 176 b) *Excerpta varia* (Frgm. Inc. Φλεγμαίνει γὰρ τὰ ἕλκεα. Expl. τῆς φύσιος τοῦ ἀνθρώπου).

Theophilus: (f. 1–94ᵛ) *Commentarius in Hippocratis aphorismos.*

Paris, Bibl. Nationale, Parisin. 2149 (?).
Same as **2149** above (*Census*: 220, nr [1064]).

De ulceribus (Frgm.).

Paris, Bibl. Nationale, Parisin. 2150; a. 1584.

Aphorismi (c. interpretat. Damascii).

Damascius, *Expositio in aphorismos Hippocratis. Sectiones VII.*

Paris, Bibl. Nationale, Parisin. 2151; s. XVI.

Erotianus: (f. 49) *Vocum Hippocraticarum conlectio* (A-O).

[Paris, Bibl. Nationale, Parisin. 2154; s. XIV].
Possibly **2144** (p. 66) or **2145** (p. 68) above (*Census*: 221, nr [1071]).

Aphorismi.

Paris, Bibl. Nationale, Parisin. 2155; s. XIV.

(f. 301^{v}) *De alimento* (Π. τροφῶν).

Paris, Bibl. Nationale, Parisin. 2161; s. XV.

Aphorismi (c. comm. Galeni).

Galenos: (f. 1) *Hippocratis aphorismi et Galeni in eos commentarii VII.*

Paris, Bibl. Nationale, Parisin. 2165; s. XVI.

(f. 1) *De morbis popularibus I et III* (pars tantum c. comm. Gal.).
(f. 1) *De morbis popularibus II. IV–VII* (pars tant., c. comm. Galeni).

Galenos: (f. 1) *In Hippocratis epidemiarum libros commentarii* (in libros III).

Paris, Bibl. Nationale, Parisin. 2166; s. XV–XVI.

(f. 89) *Praesagiorum Liber I* (c. comm. Galeni).

Galenos: (f. 89) *In Hippocratis praedictionum librum primum commentarii III.*

Paris, Bibl. Nationale, Parisin. 2168; s. XVI.

Aphorismi (c. comm. Gal.).
Prognosticon (comm. Gal.).

Galenos:
(f. 1) *Hippocratis aphorismi et Galeni in eos commentarii VII.*
(f. 172) *In Hippocratis praedictionum librum primum commentarii III.*
(f. 172) *In Hippocratis prognosticum commentarii III.*

Paris, Bibl. Nationale, Parisin. 2174; s. XVI.

(f. 1) *De morbis popularibus I et III* (L. I. III. c. c. Galeni).

Galenos:
(f. 1) *In Hippocratis epidemiarum libros commentarii* (in libr. II).
(f. 106) *In Hippocratis epidemiarum libros commentarii* (in libr. III).

Paris, Bibl. Nationale, Parisin. 2177; s. XVI.

Galenos: (f. 1) *In Hippocratis de humoribus librum commentarii III* (Frgm.).
Erotianus: (f. 96) *Vocum Hippocraticarum conlectio.*

Paris, Bibl. Nationale, Parisin. 2178; s. XIV, XV.

Aphorismi (Frgm.).
(f. 42) *De morbis hominum et remediis.*

Paris, Bibl. Nationale, Parisin. 2219; s. XV.

Aphorismi (init. mutil. Inc. οἱ ὑγιεινὰ τὰ σώματα).
(f. 105) *Prognosticon* (Frgm.).

Galenos: (f. 74) *Hippocratis aphorismi et Galeni in eos commentarii VII* (Libri II–VI, init. mutil.).

Paris, Bibl. Nationale, Parisin. 2222; s. XV.

Aphorismi (c. Meletii comm.).

Stephanus Atheniensis, *In aphorismos Hippocratis commentarius* (sub nomine Meletii).
Theophilus, *Commentarius in Hippocratis aphorismos* (Sub nomine Meletii).

(f. 104) **Meletius monachus**, *In aphorismos Hippocratis commentarius.*

Paris, Bibl. Nationale, Parisin. 2223; s. XVI.

Aphorismi (c. Meletii comm.).

Stephanus Atheniensis, *In aphorismos Hippocratis commentarius* (Apogr. *von* nr. [Parisin.] 2222 [above]).

Theophilus, *Commentarius in Hippocratis aphorismos* (*Apograph. von* [Parisin.] 2222).

Meletius monachus: (f. 158) *In aphorismos Hippocratis commentarius.*

Paris, Bibl. Nationale, Parisin. 2224; s. XIV ex., XIV–XV, XV.

Aphorismi (Frgm.).

(f. 42) **Hippokrates, Galenos**, *De urinis* (ex Gal. Hipp. etc. de urinis).

Paris, Bibl. Nationale, Parisin. 2228; s. XI, XII, XIV–XV.
See also **[2828 (? = 2228 ?)]** below (p. 87).

(f. 95) *Aphorismi* (c. comm. Theophili).

(f. 105) *Prognosticon.*

Theophilus: (f. 95–149^{v}) *Commentarius in Hippocratis aphorismos.*

Paris, Bibl. Nationale, Parisin. 2229; s. XIII, XIV.
See also **[2229 (?)]** below.

De morbis popularibus I et III (Frgm.).

(f. 25) *Hippocratis vel Dioclis epistula ad Ptolemaeum Aegypti regem.*

(f. 26) *Prognosticon.*

(f. 33) *Aphorismi* (Frgm.).

[Paris, Bibl. Nationale, Parisin. 2229 (?); s. XIII].
= ? about *De morbis popularibus*, and same as **2229** above (about *Hippocratis vel Dioclis epistula ...*) (*Census*: 229, nr [1155]).

De morbis popularibus II. IV–VII (Frgm.).

Epistula ad Ptolemaeum regem de sanitate tuenda.

[Paris, Bibl. Nationale, Parisin. 2232; s. XIV].
Possibly same as **2332** below (p. 83) (*Census*: 229–230, nr [1159]).

(f. 216) *De morbis II et III* (Frgm.).

Nationale, Bibl. Nationale, Parisin. 2240; s. XVI.
See also **[2699 (?)]** below (p. 87).

(f. 156^{v}) *Hippocratis ad Ptolemaeum regem epistula.*

[Paris, Bibl. Nationale, Parisin. 2242 (?)].
Same as **2142** above (p. 63) (*Census*: 230, nr [1168]).

De mulierum affectibus.

Paris, Bibl. Nationale, Parisin. 2247; s. XVI.
See also **[2247]** below.

De chirurgia (Exc. ex libris chirurgicis).
(f. 13) *De officina medici.*
(f. 16) *De fracturis.*
(f. 35) *De articulis.*
(f. 73^{v}) *De capitis vulneribus.*
(f. 79) *Vectiarius.*

Apollonius Citiensis, *Commentarius in Hippocratis de articulis, libri III.*
Erotianus, *Vocum Hippocraticarum conlectio.*
Galenos, *In Hippocratis de articulis librum commentarii IV.*

[Paris, Bibl. Nationale, Parisin. 2247; s. XVI].
Same as **2247** above (*Census*: 231, nr [1174]).

(f. 82) *De ossium natura.*

Paris, Bibl. Nationale, Parisin. 2248; s. XVI.
See also **[2248]** below.

(f. 18) *De officina medici.*
(f. 23^{v}) *De fracturis.*
(f. 51^{v}) *De articulis.*
(f. 105^{v}) *De capitis vulneribus.*

(f. 117) *Vectiarius.*

Apollonius Citiensis, *Commentarius in Hippocratis de articulis, libri III.*
Erotianus, *Vocum Hippocraticarum conlectio.*
Galenos, *In Hippocratis de articulis librum commentarii IV.*

[Paris, Bibl. Nationale, Parisin. 2248; s. XV].
Same as **2248** above (*Census*: 232, nr [1178]).

(f. 128) *De ossium natura.*

[Paris, Bibl. Nationale, Parisin. 2250; s. XVII].
Same as one or more of **2256**, **2258**, and **2259** below (p. 80) (*Census*: 232, nr [1180]).

Aphorismi.

Paris, Bibl. Nationale, Parisin. 2253; s. XI.
See also **[2253]** below, and **[Venedig, Bibl. S. Anton.]** below (p. 114).

(f. 1) *Prognosticon.*
(f. 37) *De diaeta (regimine) acutorum.*
(f. 34) *De alimento.*
(f. 65) *De humoribus.*
(f. 70ᵛ) *De humidorum usu.*
(f. 74ᵛ) *Epistulae* (Ἐπιβ.).
(f. 75) *De arte.*
(f. 81) *De natura hominis.*
(f. 93ᵛ) *De flatibus.*
(f. 100) *Ad Ptolemaeum regem epistula de hominis fabrica.*
(f. 100) *De locis in homine.*
(f. 117ᵛ) *De prisca medicina.*
(f. 130ᵛ) *De morbis popularibus I et III* (Lib. I et III init.).

[Paris, Bibl. Nationale, Parisin. 2253; s. XI].
Same as **2253** above (*Census*: 233, nr [1185]).

(f. –) *De salubri diaeta.*

Paris, Bibl. Nationale, Parisin. 2254; s. XV.
See also (possibly) **[2257 (?)]** below (p. 80).

De mulierum affectibus.
De natura hominis.

De septimestri partu.
(f. 1) *Index* (Indicis pars posterior Ρ-Ω).
(f. 12) *De diaeta (regimine) acutorum.*
(f. 35ᵛ) *De flatibus.*
(f. 41) *Vectiarius.*
(f. 51) *De ossium natura.*
(f. 57) *De fracturis.*
(f. 78) *De officina medici.*
(f. 82ᵛ) *De exsectione foetus. De exsectione pueri* (I).
(f. 170ᵛ) *De sterilibus.*
(f. 170ᵛ) *De superfoetatione.*
(f. 180ᵛ) *De octimestri partu.*
(f. 182) *De virginum morbis.*
(f. 183) *De natura muliebri.*
(f. 206ᵛ) *De exsectione foetus. De exsectione pueri* (II).
(f. 207ᵛ) *Praesagiorum liber I.*
(f. 207ᵛ) *Praesagiorum liber II.*
(f. 221ᵛ) *De morbo sacro.*
(f. 231ᵛ) *De fistulis.*
(f. 234ᵛ) *De haemorroïdibus.*
(f. 236ᵛ) *Coa praesagia.*
(f. 256ᵛ) *De morbis popularibus II. IV–VII.*
(f. 256ᵛ) *De morbis popularibus I et III.*
(f. 363) *Epistulae.*

Erotianus, *Vocum Hippocraticarum conlectio.*

[Paris, Bibl. Nationale, Parisin. 2254; s. XV].
Possibly same as **2255** below (*Census*: 233–234, nr [1188]).

De aëre, aquis et locis.
Prognosticon.

[Paris, Bibl. Nationale, Parisin. 2254 (?); s. XV].
Same as **2255** below (*Census*: 234, nr [1189]).

De affectionibus.
De anatome.
De arte.
De articulis.
De capitis vulneribus.
De carnibus.

De corde.
De decenti ornatu.
De dentitione.
De diebus iudicatoriis.
De genitura.
De glandulis.
De humoribus.
De humidorum usu.
De insomniis.
De internis affectionibus.
De iudicationibus.
De locis in homine.
De morbis I.
De morbis II et III.
De morbis liber IV.
De natura pueri.
De ulceribus.
De victus ratione I–III.
De visu.
Iusiurandum.
Lex.
Praeceptiones.

Paris, Bibl. Nationale, Parisin. 2255; s. XV.
See also **[1444 (?)]** (possibly) (p. 57), **[2254]** (possibly), and **[2254 (?)]** above (p. 77), and **[2255]** and **[2255 (?)]** (pp. 79) below.

(f. 1) *Index* (Indicis pars prior Α-Π).
(f. 26) *Epistulae* (Δογμ..).
(f. 55) *Iusiurandum.*
(f. 56) *Lex.*
(f. 57) *De arte.*
(f. 62v) *De prisca medicina.*
(f. 83v) *Praeceptiones.*
(f. 86v) *De medico.*
(f. 90) *De natura hominis.*
(f. 101) *De genitura.*
(f. 104v) *De natura pueri.*
(f. 119v) *De articulis.*
(f. 165) *De humoribus.*
(f. 170v) *De alimento.*

(f. 173^{v}) *De ulceribus.*
(f. 181) *De morbo sacro.*
(f. 191) *De morbis II et III.*
(f. 191) *De morbis I.*
(f. 191) *De morbis liber IV.*
(f. 265^{v}) *De affectionibus.*
(f. 281^{v}) *De internis affectionibus.*
(f. 316) *De victus ratione I–III.*
(f. 356^{v}) *De insomniis.*
(f. 361^{v}) *De visu.*
(f. 363) *De diebus iudicatoriis.*
(f. 366^{v}) *De officina medici.*
(f. 367^{v}) *De carnibus.*
(f. 369^{v}) *De anatome.*
(f. 369^{v}) *De dentitione.*
(f. 370) *De corde.*
(f. 371) *De glandulis.*
(f. 371^{v}) *Ad Ptolemaeum regem epistula de hominis fabrica.*
(f. 376) *De aëre, aquis et locis.*
(f. 378^{v}) *De humidorum usu.*
(f. 379^{v}) *De iudicationibus.*
(f. 381) *Aphorismi.*
(f. 386) *Prognosticon.*
(f. 389^{v}) *De capitis vulneribus.*
(f. 393) *De aëre, aquis et locis.*

Galenos: (f. 27) *Linguarum sive dictionum exoletarum Hippocratis explicatio.*
Soranus: (f. 53^{v}) *Hippocratis genus et vita secundum Soranum.*
Erotianus, *Vocum Hippocraticarum conlectio.*

[Paris, Bibl. Nationale, Parisin. 2255].
Same as **2255** above (*Census*: 235, nr [1191]).

De salubri diaeta.

[Paris, Bibl. Nationale, Parisin. 2255 (?)].
Same as **2255** above (*Census*: 235, nr [1192]).

De locis in homine.
De decenti ornatu.

Paris, Bibl. Nationale, Parisin. 2256; s. XIV, XV.
See also **[2250]** above (p. 76) and possibly **[2266 (?)]** below (p. 81).

De genitura (Frgm.).
(f. 9) *Aphorismi.*
(f. 23) *Prognosticon.*
(f. 83) *De mulierum affectibus.*

Paris, Bibl. Nationale, Parisin. 2257; s. XVI.
See also **[3140 (?)]** below (p. 87).

(f. 1) *Aphorismi* (c. comm. anon.).
(f. 120) *Aphorismi* (**Gal. in Aph. comm.**; des. in aph. αἱ λεπταὶ καὶ ἀκριβέες).
(f. 129) *Prognosticon* (comm. Gal.).

Galenos: (f. 129) *In Hippocratis prognosticum commentarii III.*

[Paris, Bibl. Nationale, Parisin. 2257 (?)].
Possibly same as **2254** above (p. 76) (*Census*: 235–236, nr [1195]).

De exsectione foetus. De exsectione pueri.

Paris, Bibl. Nationale, Parisin. 2258; s. XVI.
See also **[2250]** above (p. 76).

Aphorismi.

Paris, Bibl. Nationale, Parisin. 2259; s. XVI.
See also **[2250]** above (p. 76).

Aphorismi.

Paris, Bibl. Nationale, Parisin. 2260; s. XVI.

(f. 1) *Aphorismi* (c. comm. anon.; frgm.).
(f. 1750 [*sic pro* 175]) *Sententiae de vita et morte* (Expl. εἰς πεντήκοντα ἡμέρας ἀποθανεῖται).

Paris, Bibl. Nationale, Parisin. 2266; s. XIII, XIV.
See also (possibly) **[2266 (?)]** below.

Prognosticon (comm. Galeni).

(f. 93) *Aphorismi* (c. comm. Gal.).

Galenos:
(f. 1) *In Hippocratis prognosticum commentarii III.*
(f. 93) *Hippocratis aphorismi et Galeni in eos commentarii VII.*

[Paris, Bibl. Nationale, Parisin. 2266 (?)].
Possibly same as **2256** (p. 80) or **2266** above (*Census*: 236–237, nr [1206]).

Praesagiorum liber I.
Praesagiorum liber II.

Paris, Bibl. Nationale, Parisin. 2268; s. XIV, XVI.

(f. 1) *Aphorismi* (c. Gal. comm.).

Galenos, *Hippocratis aphorismi et Galeni in eos commentarii VII.*

Paris, Bibl. Nationale, Parisin. 2269; s. XV.
Also (possibly) **[2269]** below.

(f. 68) *Prognosticon.*
(f. 94) *De urinis.*
(f. 126) *De venae sectione.*

[Paris, Bibl. Nationale, Parisin. 2269].
Possibly same as **2269** above (*Census*: 237, nr [1210]).

Excerpta varia.

Paris, Bibl. Nationale, Parisin. 2276; s. XVI.

Galenos:
(f. 1) *In Hippocratis vel Polybi opus de salubri victus ratione privatorum commentarius.*
(f. 1) *In Hippocratis librum de acutorum victu commentarii IV.*

Paris, Bibl. Nationale, Parisin. 2278; s. XVI.

Aphorismi (c. comm. Gal. in fine mutil.).

Galenos: (f. 1) *Hippocratis aphorismi et Galeni in eos commentarii VII* (initio et fine mutil.).

Paris, Bibl. Nationale, Parisin. 2287; s. XV–XVI.

(f. 214^{v}) *De ulceribus.*

Galenos: (f. 191) *Linguarum sive dictionum exoletarum Hippocratis explicatio.*

Paris, Bibl. Nationale, Parisin. 2294; s. XV.

(f. 68) *De urinis.*
(f. 95^{v}–96^{v}) *Sententiae de vita et morte.*

Paris, Bibl. Nationale, Parisin. 2295; s. XIV.

Palladius, *Scholia in Hippocratis de popularibus morbis librum sextum, sectiones VIII.*

Paris, Bibl. Nationale, Parisin. 2296; s. XVI.

Aphorismi (c. comm. Theophil.).

Theophilus: (f. 1–131^{v}) *Commentarius in Hippocratis aphorismos.*
Stephanus Alexandrinus: (f. 131^{v}–277^{v}) *Scholia in Hippocratis praenotiones. Sectiones III* (*Vgl.* Costomiris, Rev. des ét. gr. II [1889] p. 356).

Paris, Bibl. Nationale, Parisin. 2301; s. XII–XIV.
See also **[2301 (?)]** below.

(f. 124) *Hippocratis vel Dioclis epistula ad Ptolemaeum Aegyptii.*

[Paris, Bibl. Nationale, Parisin. 2301 (?)].
Same as **2301** above (*Census*: 242, nr [1250]).

Ad Ptolemaeum regem epistula de hominis fabrica.

Paris, Bibl. Nationale, Parisin. 2304; s. XV.

(f. A) *De urinis* (Ex Hipp. etc. de urinis).

Paris, Bibl. Nationale, Parisin. 2308; s. XV.

(f. 12^{v}) *De urinis* (Inc. *wie im* Neapol. Bibl. dei Gerolamini [XXII. I] [p. 48]).

Paris, Bibl. Nationale, Parisin. 2315; s. XV.

(f. 282) *Ad Ptolemaeum regem epistula de hominis fabrica.*

Paris, Bibl. Nationale, Parisin. 2316; s. XV.

(f. 9) *Aphorismi* (c. comm. breviss.).
(f. 138^{v}) *De natura hominis.*
(f. 154^{v}) *Prognosticon* (Frgm.).
(f. 205) *De pulsibus* (Interrogationes et responsiones de pulsibus).
(f. 340^{v}) *De lapidum virtute.*

Paris, Bibl. Nationale, Parisin. 2317; s. XVI.

(f. 40) *De natura hominis* (Frgm.).
(f. 45) *De natura hominis* (Frgm.).

Paris, Bibl. Nationale, Parisin. 2320; s. XVI.

(f. 1) *De genitura.*
(f. 7) *Hippocratis et Galeni philosophia de natura hominis.*
(f. 13^{v}) *De venae sectione* (Περὶ τοῦ ἐκ ποίων τόπων φλεβοτομεῖν).
(f. 17^{v}) *De urinis* (Περὶ οὔρων χρηστῶν Ἱππ. καὶ Γαλ. τῶν φιλοσόφων).

Paris, Bibl. Nationale, Parisin. 2330; s. XV.
See also **[2030]** above (p. 60).

(f. 1) *Aphorismi.*
(f. 69^{v}) *Prognosticon.*

Paris, Bibl. Nationale, Parisin. 2332; s. XIV, XIV (XV), XV (XIV), XV.
See possibly **[2232]** above (p. 75), and **[2332]** below.

Prognosticon (Frgm.).
Prognosticon (Frgm.).
(f. 204^{v}) *De prisca medicina* (Frgm.).
(f. 231) *De diaeta (regimine) acutorum* (Frgm.).

Galenos :
In Hippocratis librum de acutorum victu commentarii IV (Frgm.).
Hippocratis aphorismi et Galeni in eos commentarii VII (Frgm. ex libr. I–VI).

[Paris, Bibl. Nationale, Parisin. 2332; s. XIV, XV (XIV)].
Same as **2332** above (*Census*: 244, nr [1277]).

De morbis popularibus I et III (Frgm.).
De morbis popularibus II. IV–VII (Frgm.).

(f. 204) *De arte* (Frgm.).
(f. 205ᵛ) *Praeceptiones* (Frgm.).
(f. 206) *De decenti ornatu* (Frgm.).
(f. 208) *De genitura* (Frgm.)
(f. 208) *De natura pueri* (Frgm.).
(f. 210ᵛ) *De articulis* (Frgm. »Ἐν τῷ περὶ ἄρθρων ὤμου«).
(f. 213) *De alimento* (Frgm.).
(f. 213) *De humoribus* (Frgm.).
(f. 213ᵛ) *De morbo sacro* (Frgm.).
(f. 213ᵛ) *De ulceribus* (Frgm.).
(f. 216) *De morbis I* (Frgm.).
(f. 216) *De morbis liber IV* (Frgm.).
(f. 222) *De affectionibus* (Frgm.).
(f. 223) *De internis affectionibus* (Frgm.).
(f. 224ᵛ) *De victus ratione I–III* (Frgm.).
(f. 227) *De insomniis* (Frgm.).
(f. 230) *De visu* (Frgm.).
(f. 230ᵛ) *De diebus iudicatoriis* (Frgm.).
(f. 236) *De flatibus* (Frgm.).
(f. 237) *Vectiarius* (Frgm.).
(f. 239) *De ossium natura* (Frgm.).
(f. 239ᵛ) *De fracturis* (Frgm.).
(f. 241) *De exsectione foetus. De exsectione pueri* (Frgm. I).
(f. 241) *De mulierum affectibus* (Frgm.).
(f. 248ᵛ) *De superfoetatione* (Frgm.).
(f. 249ᵛ) *De virginum morbis* (Frgm.).
(f. 250ᵛ) *De natura muliebri* (Frgm.).
(f. 251ᵛ) *Praesagiorum liber I* (Frgm.).
(f. 251ᵛ) *Praesagiorum liber II* (Frgm.).
(f. 262ᵛ) *De fistulis* (Frgm.).
(f. 262ᵛ) *De haemorroïdibus* (Frgm.).
(f. 263) *Coa praesagia* (Frgm.).
(f. 277) *Epistulae* (Frgm.).

Paris, Bibl. Nationale, Parisin. 2419; ca, a. 1460, s. XV.

(f. 153) *Jatrosophium* (Hipp. ... iatros.).
(f. 153) *De partibus hominis.*

Paris, Bibl. Nationale, Parisin. 2510; a. 1384, s. XIV.

(f. 80) **Hippokrates**, **Galenos**, **Dioscurides**, *De animalibus marinis et terrestribus ad morbos curandos idoneis.*
(f. 133ᵛ) *Remedia* (Hipp. et Gal. antidotum).

Paris, Bibl. Nationale, Parisin. 2545 (? = 2145 ? cf. Kühn l.1).
Same as **2145** above (p. 68) (*Census*: 246–247, nr [1297]).

Prognosticon.

[Paris, Bibl. Nationale, Parisin. 2545 (?) = 2145 ?].
Same as **2145** above (p. 68) (*Census*: 247, nr [1298]).

Aphorismi.
De articulis.
De fracturis.
De officina medici.
De prisca medicina.

[Paris, Bibl. Nationale, Parisin. 2545 (? = 2145 ?)].
Same as **2145** above (p. 68) (*Census*: 247–248, nr [1299]).

Coa praesagia.
De alimento.
De arte.
De articulis.
De decenti ornatu.
De diaeta (regimine) acutorum.
De diebus iudicatoriis.
De exsectione foetus. De exsectione pueri.
De humoribus.
De insomniis.
De morbis I.
De morbis II et III.
De morbis liber IV.
De morbo sacro.
De natura hominis.
De natura pueri.
De ossium natura.
De sterilibus.
De superfoetatione.
De victus ratione I–III.

De virginum morbis.
De visu.
Iusiurandum.
Lex.
Praesagiorum liber I.
Praesagiorum liber II.
Praeceptiones.
De flatibus.

[Paris, Bibl. Nationale, Parisin. 2546 (? = 2146 ?)].
Possibly same as **2146** above (p. 69) (*Census*: 248, nr [1300]).

De octimestri partu.
De septimestri partu.

Paris, Bibl. Nationale, Parisin. 2596; s. XIV.

(f. 185^{v}) *Iusiurandum.*
(f. 194) *Aphorismi* (Sect. I.; frgm.).

Soranus: (f. 184) *Hippocratis genus et vita secundum Soranum.*

Paris, Bibl. Nationale, Parisin. 2614; s. XVI.

Erotianus, *Vocum Hippocraticarum conlectio.*

Paris, Bibl. Nationale, Parisin. 2615; s. 1533 *und* 1584.

Erotianus, *Vocum Hippocraticarum conlectio.*

Paris, Bibl. Nationale, Parisin. 2651; s. XVI.

Erotianus: (f. 1) *Vocum Hippocraticarum conlectio.*

Paris, Bibl. Nationale, Parisin. 2652; s. XV.

(f. 78^{v}) *Epistulae.*

Paris, Bibl. Nationale, Parisin. 2671; s. XV.
See also **[2671 (?)]** below.

(f. 264–265^{v}) *Sententiae de vita et morte* (Sine titulo).

[Paris, Bibl. Nationale, Parisin. 2671 (?); s. XV].
Same as **2671** above (*Census*: 250, nr [1311]).

Aphorismi (c. comm. Theophil.).

[Paris, Bibl. Nationale, Parisin. 2699 (?); s. XVI].
Same as **2240** above (p. 75) (*Census*: 250, nr [1313]).

Hippocratis ad Ptolemaeum regem epistula.

Paris, Bibl. Nationale, Parisin. 2755; s. XV.

(f. 161) *Epistulae.*

[Paris, Bibl. Nationale, Parisin. 2828 (? = 2228 ?); s. –].
Same as **2228** above (p. 74) (*Census*: 251, nr [1319]).

Prognosticon.

Paris, Bibl. Nationale, Parisin. 2847; s. XVI.

(f. 139) *Excerpta varia.*

Paris, Bibl. Nationale, Parisin. 2894; s. XIII, XV–XVI.

(f. 334) *Ad Ptolemaeum regem epistula de hominis fabrica.*

Paris, Bibl. Nationale, Parisin. 3047; a. 1420.

(f. 5) *Epistulae.*

Paris, Bibl. Nationale, Parisin. 3050; s. XV.

(f. 107) *Epistulae.*

Paris, Bibl. Nationale, Parisin. 3052; s. XVI.

(f. 38) *Epistulae* (Epp. Artax. et Hipp.).

[Paris, Bibl. Nationale, Parisin. 3140 (?)].
Same as **2257** above (p. 80) (*Census*: 252–253, nr [1331]).

Aphorismi.

[Paris, Bibl. Nationale, Parisin. 3170 (?); s. –].
Same as **36** above (p. 57) (*Census*: 253, nr [1332]).

Prognosticon.

Paris, Bibl. Nationale, Suppl.
Now Paris, Bibliothèque nationale de France, supplément grec

Paris, Bibl. Nationale, Suppl. 2; s. XVI.

Galenos, *In Hippocratis de humoribus librum commentarii III.*

Paris, Bibl. Nationale, Suppl. 64; s. XV–XVII.

(f. 247) *Aphorismi* (pars comm. Theophili).

Theophilus: (f. 207–230ᵛ) *Commentarius in Hippocratis aphorismos* (Sine auctor. nomine. Expl. λειποθυμία καὶ συγκοπὴ ἕπεται. *Vgl.* Costomiris l. l. p. 357).

Paris, Bibl. Nationale, Suppl. 165; s. XV.

(f. 105) *Ad Ptolemaeum regem epistula de hominis fabrica.*

Paris, Bibl. Nationale, Suppl. 205; s. XV–XVI.

(f. 34) *Epistulae.*

Paris, Bibl. Nationale, Suppl. 270; s. XVII.

Apollonius Citiensis: (f. 351) *Commentarius in Hippocratis de articulis, libri III.*

Paris, Bibl. Nationale, Suppl. 352; s. XIII.

(f. 145ᵛ) *Epistula ad Ptolemaeum regem de sanitate tuenda.*

Paris, Bibl. Nationale, Suppl. 446; s. X.

(f. 45) *Aphorismi.*
(f. 68) *Prognosticon.*
(f. 69ᵛ) *Hippocratis ad Ptolemaeum regem epistula* (Expl. διὸ χρῶ τοῖς περιπάτοις καὶ ...).

Paris, Bibl. Nationale, Suppl. 447; s. XIV.
Vindob. med. gr. 34 ist jetzt Parisin. Suppl. 447.
See **Wien, Hofbibliothek, Vindob. med. 34** below (p. 118).

De salubri diaeta (Frgm.).
(f. 1) *Aphorismi* (c. comm. Gal.).

Galenos: (f. 1) *Hippocratis aphorismi et Galeni in eos commentarii VII.*
Galenos: (f. 229) *In Hippocratis vel Polybi opus de salubri victus ratione privatorum commentarius.*

Paris, Bibl. Nationale, Suppl. 496; s. XVII.

(f. 7–9) *Jatrosophium* (Ἰατροσόφ. ἐκ τοῦ Ἱππ. βιβλίου. Inc. Ἡ μὲν ἐν ἀρχῇ τοῦ προπάτορος δέσις. Expl. μελανόχολοι καὶ λευκόχροοι).

Paris, Bibl. Nationale, Suppl. 608; s. XVI.

(f. 178v) *Iusiurandum.*

Paris, Bibl. Nationale, Suppl. 637; s. XV.
See also (possibly) **675** below.

(f. 65) *Sententiae de vita et morte.*

Paris, Bibl. Nationale, Suppl. 675; s. XV.
Possibly same as **Suppl. 637** above (*Census*: 257, nr [1373]).

(f. 83) *Sententiae de vita et morte* (Wie im cod. monast. Ἐσφιγμένου Athos [41]).

Paris, Bibl. Nationale, Suppl. 682; s. X–XIX, XI.

(f. 85) *Aphorismi* (c. interpr. Damascii).

Damascius: (f. 85) *Expositio in aphorismos Hippocratis. Sectiones VII* (Apogr. codicis [Parisin.] 2150) (see above p. 72).

Paris, Bibl. Nationale, Suppl. 684; s. XV–XVIII.

(f. 211) *Jatrosophium* (Iatrosoph. ex Gal. Hipp. et aliis. Inc. Ἐγὼ Γαληνὸς πεπειραμένος).

Paris, Bibl. Nationale, Suppl. 688; s. XVI.

Soranus: (f. 39) *Hippocratis genus et vita secundum Soranum.*

Paris, Bibl. Nationale, Suppl. 728 (Minas IZ); s. XIV.
Same as **Suppl. 1254** below (*Census*: 258, nr [1381]).

(f. 28) *Hippocratis Ad Galenum discipulum liber de pulsibus et de temperamentis corporis humani* (*Vgl.* Costomiris Revue des ét. gr. II [1889] p. 353).

Paris, Bibl. Nationale, Suppl. 754 (Minas); s. –.
Same as **Suppl. 1254** below (*Census*: 259, nr [1382]).

(f. 523) *Hippocratis Ad Galenum discipulum liber de pulsibus et de temperamentis corporis humani* (*Vgl.* Costom. *a. a. O.* [= Revue des ét. gr. II [1889] p. 353]).

Paris, Bibl. Nationale, Suppl. 1194; s. XV.

(f. 1) *Excerpta varia.*

Paris, Bibl. Nationale, Suppl. 1254; s. XVI.
See **Suppl. 728 (Minas IZ)** and **Suppl. 754 (Minas)** above.

(f. 135) *Ad Galenum discipulum liber de pulsibus et de temperamentis corporis humani* (»Ad Gal. de pulsibus«).

Pistoia

Pistoja, Biblioteca Fabroniana, 141 (308); s. XVI.
Now Biblioteca Capitolare Fabroniana, Ms 308 (*Census*: 266, nr [1409]).

(f. 1) *Aphorismi* (c. comm. Gal.).

Galenos:
(f. 1) *Hippocratis aphorismi et Galeni in eos commentarii VII.*
(f. 146) *In Hippocratis prognosticum commentarii III.*

Rom, Bibl. Angelica
Roma, Biblioteca Angelica

Rom, Bibl. Angelica, 4 (C 4.16); s. XVI in.
Now Ang. gr. 4 (*Census*: 270, nr [1418]).

(f. 171) *De quattuor elementis et humoribus naturae hominis* (Inc. Ἰστέον ἐστιν· ὁ ἄνθρωπος ἐπίσταται [sic!]. Expl. ὅσα δὲ γένηται ἐν χειμῶν⟨ι⟩ ἀπαλλάσσονται).
(f. 172) *Ad Ptolemaeum regem epistula de hominis fabrica* (Expl. *wie im* Monacens. 72 [above p. 46]).
(f. 174) *De sensibus* (Frgm. Inc. Αἰσθητήρια δέ ἐστιν ἐν τῷ ἀνθρώπῳ. Expl. καὶ ξηρᾶς κράσεώς εἰσιν).

Rom, Bibl. Angelica, 80 (C.1. 11); s. XV.
Now Ang. gr. 80 (*Census*: 271, nr [1421]).

(f. 233) *Aphorismi*.

Rom, Bibl. Barberin.
Now at Città del Vaticano, Biblioteca Apostolica Vaticana, *Barberiniani*

Rom, Bibl. Barberin., I 5; s. XV.
Now *Vaticanus Barberinianus graecus* 5 (*Census*: 272, nr [1422]).

(f. 1) *Aphorismi* (c. comm. Gal.; Expl. θανάσιμον τὸ τοιοῦτον).
(f. 237v) *De aëre, aquis et locis*.

Rom, Bibl. Barberin., I 11 (= 136); s. XVI.
Now *Vaticanus Barberinianus graecus* 11 (*Census*: 272, nr [1423]).
See also **136 (= I 11)** below.

(f. 2) *Aphorismi*.

Rom, Bibl. Barberin., I 127; s. XVI.
Now *Vaticanus Barberinianus graecus* 127 (*Census*: 273, nr [1431]).
See also (possibly) **276** below.

(f. 250v) *De mulieribus* (Inscr. Περὶ διαγνώσεως τῶν κυϊσκουσῶν γυναικῶν καὶ περὶ τῶν ἐν γαστρὶ ἐχουσῶν).
(f. 310) *Hippocratis vel Dioclis epistula ad Ptolemaeum Aegyptii regem*.
(f. 313) *De insomniis*.

(f. 336) *Excerpta varia* (Inc. Μετὰ τὸ Πυθαγόραν. Expl. τέθνηκάς μοι).

Rom, Bibl. Barberin., III 63 (= 245); s. XVI.
Now *Vaticanus Barberinianus graecus* 344 (*Census*: 273, nr [1434]).

(f. 394–414ᵛ) **Hippokrates, Galenos, Meletius monachus**, *Jatrosophium* (Ἰατροσόφιον ἐκλελεγμένον Γαλ. Ἱππ. καὶ Μελετίου περὶ γυναικός. Expl. εἰς τὰ νευροχαλαστικά).

Rom, Bibl. Barberin., 136 (= I 11); s. XVI.
Same as **I 11 (136)** above.
= *Vaticanus Barberinianus graecus* 11 (*Census*: 273, nr [1437]).

(f. 47) *Prognosticon*.

Rom, Bibl. Barberin., 276; s. – (?).
Possibly same **as I 127** above.
= ? *Vaticanus Barberinianus graecus* 127 (*Census*: 273, nr [1438]).

Opera varia.

Rom, Bibl. Corsiniana (= Acc. d. Lincei)
Now Roma, Biblioteca Corsiniana, Accademia dei Lincei

Rom, Bibl. Corsiniana (= Acc. d. Lincei), 1410 (36. E. 26); s. –.
Now *Corsin.* 36.E.26 (1410) (*Census*: 274, nr [1441]).

(f. 343) *Prognosticon* (Inc. Εἰ δὲ κεφαλαλγίαν ἔχει ἢ οἴδημα).
(f. 344) *Remedia* (Ἀλάτιον Ἱππ.).
(f. 348ᵛ) *De morbo sacro* (Inc. Μέλλοντας ἡμᾶς ἄρχεσθαι περὶ φύσεως ἀνθρώπου).

Rom, Bibl. Vallicellana
Roma, Biblioteca Vallicelliana

Rom, Bibl. Vallicellana, 78 (F 9); s. XVI.
Now F 9 (*Census*: 276, nr [1447]).

Erotianus: (f. 188–196ᵛ) *Vocum Hippocraticarum conlectio* (Expl. παρὰ τὸ δόρυ^ει παύειν · ὃ γὰρ ἡμεῖς).

Rom, Bibl. Vallicellana, 1106 (F 83); s. XV–XVI.
Now F 83 (*Census*: 276, nr [1448]).

(f. 188v–190) *De insomniis* (Expl. ἡ ταραχή).

Rom, Bibl. Vaticana, Ottobon.
Now Città del Vaticano, Biblioteca Apostolica Vaticana, *Ottoboniani*

Rom, Bibl. Vaticana, Ottobon. 150; s. XVI.

(f. 47) *Aphorismi*.

Rom, Bibl. Vaticana, Ottobon. 157 A; s. XVI.

(f. 1) *Aphorismi*.

Rom, Bibl. Vaticana, Ottobon. 157 B; s. XV.

(f. 1) *Aphorismi*.
(f. 23v) *Prognosticon*.

Rom, Bibl. Vaticana, Ottobon. 192; s. XVI–XVII.

(f. 16) *Prognosticon* (Frgm. Inc. Εἰσὶ δὲ τὰ δώδεκα ζώδια).

Rom, Bibl. Vaticana, Palat.
Now Città del Vaticano, Biblioteca Apostolica Vaticana, *Palatini*

Rom, Bibl. Vaticana, Palat. 126; s. XVI.

(f. 242) *Excerpta varia*.

Rom, Bibl. Vaticana, Palat. 128; s. XV.

(f. 26v) *Aphorismi* (aphorismi XIV priores c. Gal. comm.).

Galenos: (f. 26v) *Hippocratis aphorismi et Galeni in eos commentarii VII* (in aph. XIV primos).

Rom, Bibl. Vaticana, Palat. 129; s. XV.

(f. 49) *Excerpta varia*.

Rom, Bibl. Vaticana, Palat. 132; s. XV.

(f. 215^{v}) *Epistulae* (Epp. 14).

Rom, Bibl. Vaticana, Palat. 143; s. XV.

(f. 137) *Prognosticon.*
(f. 150) *Aphorismi* (Libri I–III et V in fine mutil.).
(f. 158) *De urinis.*
(f. 162) *De sudoribus* (De sudoribus febriculosis).

Galenos: (f. 164) *De victus ratione in morbis acutis ex Hippocratis sententia* (Inc. Μελίκρητον δὲ πινόμενον. »Spectare videntur ad Gal. libr. de victus ratione in morb. acut., ex Hipp. sententia.«).

Rom, Bibl. Vaticana, Palat. 155; s. XVI.

(f. 119^{v}) *Hippocratis ad Ptolemaeum regem epistula.*

Rom, Bibl. Vaticana, Palat. 157; s. XIV.

Galenos: (f. 2 [= 2v]) *In Hippocratis prognosticum commentarii IIII.*

Rom, Bibl. Vaticana, Palat. 173; s. XV.
= ? *Vaticanus Reginensis* 173 below (p. 96) (*Census*: 279, nr [1474]).

Galenos: (f. 1) *In Hippocratis prognosticum commentarii III.*

Rom, Bibl. Vaticana, Palat. 192; s. XV.

(f. 1) *Iusiurandum.*
(f. 1^{v}) *Aphorismi* (Aph. ult. Περὶ ἐγκεφάλου ἐσφακελισμένου).
(f. 9) *Prognosticon* (Lib. I et II).
(f. 13^{v}) *De diaeta (regimine) acutorum* (Πρὸς τὰς Κνιδίας γνώμας ἢ περὶ πτισάνης).
(f. 18) *De aquis* (De aqua et balneo).
(f. 18^{v}) *De morbis I.*
(f. 18^{v}) *De morbis II et III.*
(f. 18^{v}) *De morbis liber IV.*
(f. 23^{v}) *De officina medici.*
(f. 25) *De medico.*
(f. 26) *De aëre, aquis et locis.*
(f. 30) *De anatome.*
(f. 30 [*nach*]) *De dentitione.*

(f. 31) *De sterilibus.*
(f. 36) *De superfoetatione.*
(f. 39ᵛ) *De exsectione foetus. De exsectione pueri* (II ?).
(f. 40) *De iudicationibus.*
(f. 41ᵛ) *De corde.*
(f. 42ᵛ) *De carnibus.*
(f. 45ᵛ) *De glandulis.*
(f. 47) *De locis in homine.*
(f. 54ᵛ) *De fracturis.*
(f. 56ᵛ) *De pede.*
(f. 57) *De calce.*
(f. 64) *De capitis vulneribus.*
(f. 71) *De articulis.*
(f. 91) *De natura hominis.*
(f. 95) *De natura pueri.*
(f. 101) *De genitura.*
(f. 102ᵛ) *De septimestri partu.*
(f. 103) *De octimestri partu.*
(f. 104ᵛ) *De virginum morbis.*
(f. 105) *De natura muliebri.*
(f. 114) *De morbis popularibus I et III.*
(f. 114) *De morbis popularibus II. IV–VII.*
(f. 153) *De mulierum affectibus* (Lib. I fine mutil.).
(f. 171) *Epistulae.*

Rom, Bibl. Vaticana, Palat. 199; s. XIII.

(f. 18) *Prognosticon.*
(f. 39 [so !]) *Prognosticon.*
(f. 44 [so !]) *Aphorismi.*
(f. 47) *Aphorismi* (c. comm.).

Rom, Bibl. Vaticana, Palat. 278; s. XIV–XV.

Galenos: (f. 31ᵛ) *Hippocratis aphorismi et Galeni in eos commentarii VII* (in sectiones VI).

Rom, Bibl. Vaticana, Palat. 279; s. XIV–XV.

(f. 1) *Aphorismi* (sectt. duae primae c. scholiis).
(f. 31ᵛ) *Aphorismi* (sectt. duae primae c. scholiis; sectiones VI c. comm. Galeni).

Rom, Bibl. Vaticana, Palat. 297; s. XV–XVI.

Aphorismi (Liber VII c. scholiis anon.).
(f. 157v) *Remedia* (de remediis ad partum proficientibus. Inscr. Κυητήριον Ἱππ.).

Rom, Bibl. Vaticana, Palat. 363; s. XV.

(f. 108) *Ad Galenum discipulum liber de pulsibus et de temperamentis corporis humani.*

Rom, Bibl. Vaticana, Palat. 385; s. XV–XVI.

Galenos: (f. 1) *Hippocratis aphorismi et Galeni in eos commentarii VII* (init. et fine mutil.).

Rom, Bibl. Vaticana, Palat. 398; s. X.

(f. 282) *Epistulae* (Epp. 1–24 ?).

Rom, Bibl. Vaticana, Palat. 400; s. XV.

(f. 171) *Excerpta varia* (Inc. Ὅταν ἀκμάζῃ τὸ νόσημα).
(f. 399) *Remedia* (De prophylacticis adversus arthriticos affectus ex Hippocrate Galeno aliisque).

Rom, Bibl. Vaticana, Palat. 428; s. XV–XVI, XV–XVII.

(f. 1) *Index* (Index in Gal., Alex. Aphr. et Hipp. aliquot opuscola).

Rom, Bibl. Vaticana, Reg. Suec.
Now Città del Vaticano, Biblioteca Apostolica Vaticana, *Reginenses*

Rom, Bibl. Vaticana, Reg. Suec. 173; s. XV.
See also (possibly) **Palat. 173** above (p. 94).

Galenos:
(f. 73v) *In Hippocratis librum de acutorum victu commentarii IV.*
(f. 185) *Galeni in Hippocratis de natura hominis lib. commentarii II.*
(f. 222) *In Hippocratis vel Polybi opus de salubri victus ratione privatorum commentarius.*

Rom, Bibl. Vaticana, Reg. Suec. 175; s. XIV.

Galenos:
(f. 1 [= 2r]) *In Hippocratis prognosticum commentarii III.*
(f. 89) *In Hippocratis praedictionum librum primum commentarii III.*

Rom, Bibl. Vaticana, Reg. Suec. 181; a. 1364.

(f. 281v *und* f. 283) *Ad Ptolemaeum regem epistula de hominis fabrica* (Frgm. Inc f. 281v: Ὁ ἄνθρωπος διαιρεῖται; f. 283: Ἀπὸ μηνὸς Νοεμβρίου).

Rom, Bibl. Vaticana, Reg. Suec. 182; s. XV.

(f. 16) *Iusiurandum.*
(f. 16v) *De febribus* (Inc. *wie im* Leydens. Voss. [fol. 10]) (p. 32).
(f. 18) *De salubri diaeta* (Frgm. Inscr. *und* Inc. *wie im* Monac. 71) (p. 45).
(f. 20v) *De genitura.*
(f. 34) *De natura pueri.*
(f. 40) *De urinis.*
(f. 41v) *De pulsibus* (Inc. Ἥκω δή σοι καὶ τὸ περὶ).
(f. 43v. 45v) *De febribus* (Inc. *wie im* Parisin. 1884) (p. 59).
(f. 48) *Ad Ptolemaeum regem epistula de hominis fabrica* (»de partibus corp. hum.; frgm. initio mutilum.« Inc. Λέγεται δὲ καὶ γαστήρ, ὅτε περιαγής ἐστιν).
(f. 57v) *De victus ratione I–III* (fine mutil.).
(f. 58) *Aphorismi* (sectio prima).
(f. 60) *Ad Ptolemaeum regem epistula de hominis fabrica* (»de part. corp. hum.« Inc. Συνέστηκεν ὁ ἄνθρωπος).
(f. 83) *De morbis I* (Frgm.).
(f. 83) *De morbis II et III.*
(f. 83) *De morbis liber IV.*

Rom, Bibl. Vaticana, Urbin.
Now Città del Vaticano, Biblioteca Apostolica Vaticana, *Urbinates*

Rom, Bibl. Vaticana, Urbin. 64; s. X–XI, XIII.

(f. 1) *Aphorismi.*
(f. 96) *Prognosticon.*
(f. 100) *De flatibus* (Frgm.).

(f. 100–103) *Excerpta varia* (I. Ἐκ τοῦ π. φυσῶν. II. Π. χειρουργίας. III. Π. ἀφανῶν νοσημάτων. IV. Τὸ δι' ἐναντίων συγγίνεται ἡ ἰατρική).
(f. 102) *De remediis.*
f. 104) *Epistulae.*
(f. 116) *Iusiurandum* (Frgm. »ἐκ τοῦ κατὰ τὸν Ἱππ. ὅρκου, καθ' ὅσον οἷόν τε Χριστιανῷ ὀμόσαι«).

Galenos (*Ist der Commentar des* Palladius *unter den Namen des* Galen): (f. 48v) *Scholia in Hippocratis de popularibus morbis librum sextum, sectiones VIII* (Σχόλιον τῆς ἕκτης ἐπιδημίας ἀπὸ φωνῆς Γαλ. VII partes. Inc. Ἄρτι ταῖς μεθόδοις τὰ ὀξέα τῶν νοσημάτων).
Palladius (sub Galeni nomine): (f. 94) *Scholia in Hippocratis de popularibus morbis librum sextum, sectiones VIII.*

Rom, Bibl. Vaticana, Urbin. 65; s. XIV.

Galenos: (f. 1) *Hippocratis aphorismi et Galeni in eos commentarii VII.*

Rom, Bibl. Vaticana, Urbin. 67; s. XIII, XIV, XIV–XV, XV.

Galenos: (f. 33) *In Hippocratis de humoribus librum commentarii III.*

Rom, Bibl. Vaticana, Urbin. 68; s. XIV.

(f. 4) *Iusiurandum.*
(f. 4) *Lex.*
(f. 7) *De arte.*
(f. 17) *Esse re vera artes.*
(f. 17v) *De substantia artis medicae. Definitio artis medicae.*
(f. 20) *De prisca medicina.*
(f. 26v) *Praeceptiones.*
(f. 28v) *De decenti ornatu.*
(f. 30) *De natura hominis.*
(f. 35) *De salubri diaeta* (Frgm.).
(f. 35) *De genitura.*
(f. 38v) *De natura pueri.*
(f. 38v) *De articulis.*
(f. 72) *De humoribus.*
(f. 74v) *De alimento.*
(f. 76v) *De ulceribus.*
(f. 80v) *De morbo sacro.*
(f. 86v) *De morbis I.*

(f. 86v) *De morbis II et III.*
(f. 86v) *De morbis liber IV.*
(f. 91) *De natura hominis.*
(f. 138) *De internis affectionibus.*
(f. 159) *De victus ratione I–III.*
(f. 183) *De insomniis.*
(f. 186) *De visu.*
(f. 187) *De diebus iudicatoriis.*
(f. 189) *Aphorismi* (Sectio I–VI).
(f. 201v) *Prognosticon.*
(f. 209v) *De diaeta (regimine) acutorum.*
(f. 225) *De flatibus.*
(f. 229) *Vectiarius.*
(f. 237v) *De ossium natura.*
(f. 240) *De fracturis.*
(f. 255) *De officina medici.*
(f. 257) *De exsectione foetus. De exsectione pueri* (I).
(f. 258v) *De mulierum affectibus.*
(f. 308v) *De sterilibus.*
(f. 315) *De superfoetatione.*
(f. 319v) *De septimestri partu.*
(f. 321v) *De octimestri partu.*
(f. 322v) *De virginum morbis.*
(f. 323) *De natura muliebri.*
(f. 337) *De exsectione foetus. De exsectione pueri* (II).
(f. 337v) *Praesagiorum liber I.*
(f. 337v) *Praesagiorum liber II.*
(f. 351v) *De fistulis.*
(f. 353v) *De haemorroïdibus.*
(f. 354v) *Coa praesagia.*
(f. 360v) *De morbis popularibus I et III.*
(f. 360v) *De morbis popularibus II. IV–VII.*
(f. 418v) *Epistulae.*

Galenos: (f. 3) *Linguarum sive dictionum exoletarum Hippocratis explicatio.*
Soranus: (f. 4) *Hippocratis genus et vita secundum Soranum.*
Galenos: (f. 26v) *Scholion in Hippocratis* Παραγγελίας.
Erotianus, *Vocum Hippocraticarum conlectio.*

Rom, Bibl. Vaticana, Vatic.
Now Città del Vaticano, Biblioteca Apostolica Vaticana, *Vaticani graeci*

[Rom, Bibl. Vaticana, Vatic. 216].
= ? **278** below (p. 102) (*Census*: 289, nr [1519]).

De flatibus.
De ossium natura.

Rom, Bibl. Vaticana, Vatic. 276; s. XII.

(f. 1) *Laterculi antiqui.*
(f. 1) *Iusiurandum.*
(f. 1^{v}) *Aphorismi.*
(f. 1^{v}) *Lex.*
(f. 9^{v}) *Prognosticon.*
(f. 14^{v}) *De diaeta (regimine) acutorum.*
(f. 26^{v}) *De officina medici.*
(f. 27^{v}) *De fracturis.*
(f. 37^{v}) *De articulis.*
(f. 57) *De capitis vulneribus.*
(f. 63^{v}) *De aëre, aquis et locis.*
(f. 67^{v}) *De morbis popularibus II. IV–VII.*
(f. 67^{v}) *De morbis popularibus I et III.*
(f. 107) *De natura hominis.*
(f. 111^{v}) *De natura pueri.*
(f. 112) *De septimestri partu.*
(f. 117^{v}) *De genitura.*
(f. 119) *De superfoetatione.*
(f. 122^{v}) *De octimestri partu.*
(f. 124) *De virginum morbis.*
(f. 124^{v}) *De natura muliebri.*
(f. 133) *De dentitione.*
(f. 134) *De locis in homine.*
(f. 141^{v}) *De mulierum affectibus.*
(f. 169^{v}) *De anatome.*
(f. 178^{v}) *De sterilibus.*
(f. 184^{v}) *De superfoetatione.*
(f. 187^{v}) *De exsectione foetus. De exsectione pueri* (II).
(f. 188) *De medico.*
(f. 189^{v}) *De iudicationibus.*

(f. 191) *De corde.*
(f. 192) *De carnibus.*
(f. 195) *De glandulis.*
(f. 196ᵛ) *Epistulae.*

Rom, Bibl. Vaticana, Vatic. 277; s. XIV.

(f. 11) *Laterculi antiqui.*
(f. 25) *Iusiurandum.*
(f. 25ᵛ) *Lex.*
(f. 26) *De arte.*
(f. 29ᵛ) *De prisca medicina.*
(f. 37ᵛ) *Praeceptiones.*
(f. 40) *De decenti ornatu.*
(f. 49ᵛ) *De genitura.*
(f. 52) *De natura pueri.*
(f. 43) *De natura hominis.*
(f. 61) *De articulis.*
(f. 91) *De humoribus.*
(f. 95) *De alimento.*
(f. 97) *De ulceribus.*
(f. 102) *De morbo sacro.*
(f. 109) *De morbis I.*
(f. 109) *De morbis II et III.*
(f. 109) *De morbis liber IV.*
(f. 155ᵛ) *De affectionibus.*
(f. 166) *De internis affectionibus.*
(f. 187) *De victus ratione I–III.*
(f. 211ᵛ) *De insomniis.*
(f. 214) *De visu.*
(f. 215ᵛ) *De diebus iudicatoriis.*
(f. 217) *Aphorismi.*
(f. 227ᵛ) *Prognosticon.*
(f. 234ᵛ) *De diaeta (regimine) acutorum.*
(f. 250ᵛ) *De flatibus.*
(f. 254) *Vectiarius.*
(f. 260ᵛ) *De ossium natura.*
(f. 265) *De fracturis.*
(f. 279ᵛ) *De officina medici.*
(f. 282ᵛ) *De mulierum affectibus.*
(f. 282) *De exsectione foetus. De exsectione pueri* (I).

(f. 338ᵛ) *De sterilibus.*
(f. 347ᵛ) *De superfoetatione.*
(f. 351ᵛ) *De septimestri partu.*
(f. 353ᵛ) *De octimestri partu.*
(f. 355) *De virginum morbis.*
(f. 355ᵛ) *De natura muliebri.*
(f. 372) *De exsectione foetus. De exsectione pueri* (II).
(f. 372ᵛ) *Praesagiorum liber I.*
(f. 372ᵛ) *Praesagiorum liber II.*
(f. 387) *De fistulis.*
(f. 389ᵛ) *De haemorroïdibus.*
(f. 390ᵛ) *Coa praesagia.*
(f. 397) *De morbis popularibus I et III.*
(f. 397ᵛ) *De morbis popularibus II. IV–VII.*
(f. 462) *Epistulae.*

Erotianus: (f. 2) *Vocum Hippocraticarum conlectio.*
Galenos: (f. 12) *Linguarum sive dictionum exoletarum Hippocratis explicatio.*
Soranus: (f. 24) *Hippocratis genus et vita secundum Soranum.*

Rom, Bibl. Vaticana, Vatic. 278; a. 1512.
See also **[Vatic. 216]** above (possibly) (p. 100).

(f. 27ᵛ) *Iusiurandum.*
(f. 28) *Lex.*
(f. 29) *De arte.*
(f. 30) *De prisca medicina* (Inscr. περὶ ὑπάρξεως ἰητρικῆς· ὅρος ἰητρικός).
(f. 30) *De substantia artis medicae. Definitio artis medicae.*
(f. 54ᵛ) *De decenti ornatu.*
(f. 50ᵛ) *Praeceptiones.*
(f. 59) *De natura hominis.*
(f. 64ᵛ) *De humoribus.*
(f. 70ᵛ) *De victus ratione I–III* (Frgm.).
(f. 75) *De genitura.*
(f. 80ᵛ) *De natura pueri.*
(f. 103) *De articulis.*
(f. 170) *De alimento.*
(f. 173) *De ulceribus.*
(f. 183) *De morbo sacro.*
(f. 196ᵛ) *De morbis I.*
(f. 196ᵛ) *De morbis II et III.*

(f. 196^{v}) *De morbis liber IV.*
(f. 298^{v}) *De affectionibus.*
(f. 320) *De internis affectionibus.*
(f. 370) *De victus ratione I–III.*
(f. 426) *De insomniis.*
(f. 434) *De visu.*
(f. 436^{v}) *De diebus iudicatoriis.*
(f. 441) *Aphorismi.*
(f. 466) *Prognosticon.*
(f. 480^{v}) *De diaeta (regimine) acutorum.*
(f. 520) *De flatibus.*
(f. 528^{v}) *Vectiarius.*
(f. 542^{v}) *De ossium natura.*
(f. 552) *De fracturis.*
(f. 584) *De officina medici.*
(f. 589 *und* –) *De exsectione foetus. De exsectione pueri* (I. II).
(f. 591^{v}) *De mulierum affectibus.*
(f. 699^{v}) *De sterilibus.*
(f. 717) *De superfoetatione.*
(f. 727^{v}) *De septimestri partu* (Inc. *und* Expl. *wie im* Holkham nr. 282) (p. 26).
(f. 733) *De octimestri partu.*
(f. 735) *De virginum morbis.*
(f. 736^{v}) *De natura muliebri.*
(f. 773^{v}) *Praesagiorum liber I.*
(f. 773^{v}) *Praesagiorum liber II.*
(f. 808) *De haemorroïdibus.*
(f. 803^{v}) *De fistulis.*
(f. 810^{v}) *Coa praesagia.*
(f. 824^{v}) *De morbis popularibus I et III.*
(f. 824^{v}) *De morbis popularibus II. IV–VII.*
(f. 965) *Epistulae.*

Soranus: (f. 25^{v}) *Hippocratis genus et vita secundum Soranum.*

Rom, Bibl. Vaticana, Vatic. 279; s. –, XII.
Verbleib unbekannt.
See *Census*: 290–291, nr [1524].

(f. 95) *Aphorismi* (**c. comm. Theophil.**).

Galenos: (f. 31) *Hippocratis aphorismi et Galeni in eos commentarii VII.*

Rom, Bibl. Vaticana, Vatic. 280; s. XV.

(f. 154ᵛ) *Aphorismi.*

Galenos: (f. 1) *Hippocratis aphorismi et Galeni in eos commentarii VII.*

Rom, Bibl. Vaticana, Vatic. 283; s. XIV.

(f. 4) *Prognosticon.*
(f. 9) *Praesagiorum liber I.*
(f. 9) *Praesagiorum liber II.*

Galenos: (f. 22) *Hippocratis aphorismi et Galeni in eos commentarii VII.*

Rom, Bibl. Vaticana, Vatic. 285; s. XV.

(f. 287) *Hippocratis ad Galenum discipulum liber de pulsibus et de temperamentis corporis humani* (Ἱ. πρ. Γαλ. ... π. διπλάσεως ἀνθρώπου).

Rom, Bibl. Vaticana, Vatic. 293; s. XVI.

(f. 219) *Hippocratis ad Ptolemaeum regem epistula.*

Rom, Bibl. Vaticana, Vatic. 294; s. –.

(f. 70ᵛ) *Prognosticon* (»Διαγνωστικά«).
(f. 88ᵛ) *De diaeta (regimine) acutorum.*
(f. 106ᵛ) *Aphorismi.*

Rom, Bibl. Vaticana, Vatic. 690; s. XV.

(f. 257ᵛ) *Hippocratis ad Ptolemaeum regem epistula.*

Rom, Bibl. Vaticana, Vatic. 876; s. XV.

(f. 4) *Hippocratis ad Ptolemaeum regem epistula.*

Rom, Bibl. Vaticana, Vatic. 1062; s. XVI.

Theophilus: (f. 1) *Commentarius in Hippocratis aphorismos.*

Rom, Bibl. Vaticana, Vatic. 1063; s. XIII.

Galenos: (f. 1) *In Hippocratis prognosticum commentarii III* (Der Anfang des Commentars ist verloren gegangen. Anfang = K. XVIII B 46).

Rom, Bibl. Vaticana, Vatic. 1065; s. XIII.

(f. 98) *Hippocratis ad Ptolemaeum regem epistula.*

Rom, Bibl. Vaticana, Vatic. 1066; s. XVI.
s. XV.

(f. 7^{v}) *Ad Ptolemaeum regem epistula de hominis fabrica.*

Rom, Bibl. Vaticana, Vatic. 1095; s. XV.

(f. 279^{v}) *Hippocratis ad Ptolemaeum regem epistula.*

Rom, Bibl. Vaticana, Vatic. 1133 (1134 Kl.); s. –, XVII.
= *Vaticanus graecus* 1133 (*Census*: 298, nr [1565]).

(f. 53) *De remediis.*

Erotianus, *Vocum Hippocraticarum conlectio* (Apogr. codicis [*Vat. gr.*] 277 [above p. 101]).

Rom, Bibl. Vaticana, Vatic. 1276; s. XIII.

(f. 180) *Ad Ptolemaeum regem epistula de hominis fabrica* (*Vielleicht diselbe Epist. wie im* Vatic. 1066 [above]).

Rom, Bibl. Vaticana, Vatic. 1309; s. XVI.

(f. 302^{v}) *Epistulae.*

Rom, Bibl. Vaticana, Vatic. 1354; s. XVI.

(f. 92^{v}) *Epistulae.*

Rom, Bibl. Vaticana, Vatic. 1467; s. XV–XVI.

(f. 140) *Epistulae* (Epp. praecip. Hipp. et Democr.).

Rom, Bibl. Vaticana, Vatic. 1759; s. XV (XVII ?).

(f. 235^{v}) *De genitura* (Frgm. Inc. Νόμος μέν. Expl. ἔξωθεν σαρκώδεις).

Rom, Bibl. Vaticana, Vatic. 1858; s. –.

Galenos: (f. 234) *In Hippocratis prognosticum commentarii III* (Inc. Ὅτι μὲν ἀντί. Expl. εὐθέως ὁμολογουμένου ὡς τα ...).

Rom, Bibl. Vaticana, Vatic. 1879; s. XV.

Soranus: (f. 159) *Hippocratis genus et vita secundum Soranum.*

Rom, Bibl. Vaticana, Vatic. 2154; s. XVI.

Damascius: (f. 3) *Expositio in Prognostica Hippocratis. Sectiones II.*

Rom, Bibl. Vaticana, Vatic. 2238; s. XV.

(f. 180) *Iusiurandum.*

Rom, Bibl. Vaticana, Vatic. 2254; s. X–XI.

(f. 21) *Prognosticon* (Init. mutil.).

Theophilus: (f. 25) *Commentarius in Hippocratis aphorismos* (Sine auctor. nomine. Expl. καὶ οἷον ὑποχόνδρια μετέωρα = Dtz. II 500, 2).

Rom, Bibl. Vaticana, Vatic. 2304 [olim 2217]; s. XV, XV–XVI.
Now *Vaticanus graecus* 2304 (*Census*: 306, nr [1603]).

(f. 1) *Iusiurandum.*

Sens

Sens, Bibl. communale, Miscell. 187; s. XVII.
Now Bibliothèque municipale, 187 (*Census*: 312, nr [1616]).
Printed edition (Paris, 1560) with Latin handwritten marginal notes.

(f. 328) *Prognosticon* (Frgm.).

Tübingen

Tübingen, Univ.-Bibl., 23; s. XVI.
Now Mb23 (*Census*: 316, nr [1619]).

De humoribus (Frgm. **Scholia** in Hipp. π. χυμῶν).

Tübingen, Univ.-Bibl., 37; a. 1584.
Now Mb 37 (*Census*: 316, nr [1620]).

(nr. 13) *De humoribus* (Frgm. *Wie im* Tubing. 23).

Turin, Bibl. Nazionale (Universitaria)
Now Torino, Biblioteca Nazionale Universitaria

Turin, Bibl. Nazionale (Universitaria), Taurin. 156 b II 10; s. XVI.
Now C. VI. 10 (*Census*: 319, nr [1627]).

(f. 115^{v}) *Prognosticon* (Frgm.).

Turin, Bibl. Nazionale (Universitaria), Taurin. 177 b II 31; s. XVI.
Verbrannt.
Now B. V. 16 (*Census*: 319, nr [1628]).
This manuscript has not been destroyed.

(f. 33) *Epistula ad Ptolemaeum regem de sanitate tuenda.*

Turin, Bibl. Nazionale (Universitaria), Taurin. 179 b II 33; s. XVI.
Durch Feuer stark beschädigt.
Now B. V. 33 (*Census*: 319, nr [1629]).
See also **B V 33 (179 b II 33)** below.

(f. 48^{v}) *Excerpta varia.*

Turin, Bibl. Nazionale (Universitaria), Taurin. 287 c I 42; s. XV.
Durch Feuer stark beschädigt.
Now C. VI. 3 (*Census*: 319, nr [1630]).
See also **C VI 3 (287 c I 42)** below.

(f. 201) *Hippocratis vel Dioclis epistula ad Ptolemaeum Aegyptii regem.*

Turin, Bibl. Nazionale (Universitaria), Taurin. B V 33 (179 b II 33); s. XVI.
Durch Feuer stark beschädigt.
Now B. V. 33 (*Census*: 320, nr [1632]).
See also **179 b II 33** above.

(f. 326) *Aphorismi.*

Turin, Bibl. Nazionale (Universitaria), Taurin. C VI 3 (287 c I 42); s. XV.
Durch Feuer stark beschädigt.
= C. VI. 3 (*Census*: 320, nr [1633]).
See also **287 c I 42** above.

(f. 199) *Ad Galenum discipulum liber de pulsibus et de temperamentis corporis humani* (»Ad Gal. suum discip. epistolium quoddam de corpore humano, necnon elementorum brevis expositio«).
(f. 201) *Hippocratis vel Dioclis epistula ad Ptolemaeum Aegyptii regem.*

Turin, Bibl. Nazionale (Universitaria), Taurin. C VI 21 (b VI 18); s. XVI.
= C. VI. 21 (*Census*: 320, nr [1634]).

(f. 26[v]) *Prognostica* (Π. καιρῶν πρόγνωσις).

Upsala, Upsal. bibl. acad.
Now Uppsala Universitet

Upsala, Upsal. bibl. acad., 8 (e don. Jo. Gabr. Sparfwenf. 49); s. –, XV.
Now Gr 8 (*Census*: 320, nr [1635]).

(f. 99) *Epistulae* (Epp. 8. 9. 1).

Upsala, Upsal. bibl. acad., 34; s. XV–XVI.
Now Gr 34 (*Census*: 321, nr [1638]).

Theophilus: (f. 2) *Commentarius in Hippocratis aphorismos* (Expl. νομίζειν ἀνίατα).

Venedig, Bibl. Nazionale Marciana, Marcian.
Now Venezia, Biblioteca Nazionale Marciana, *Marciani graeci*

[Venedig, Bibl. Nazionale Marciana, Marcian.].
= ? *graecus* 269 (coll. 533) below (p. 109) (*Census*: 327, nr [1653]).

Coa praesagia.
Praesagiorum liber II.

[Venedig, Bibl. Nazionale Marciana, Marcian.].
Possibly *graecus* 269 (coll. 533) below (*Census*: 327, nr [1654]).

Galenos, *In librum Hippocratis de aetatum aegritudinibus.*

[Venedig, Bibl. Nazionale Marciana, Marcian. ?].
Possibly *graecus* 269 (coll. 533) below (*Census*: 328, nr [1656]).

Praesagiorum liber II.

[Venedig, Bibl. Nazionale Marciana, Marcian. ap. Montf. I 472].
= ? *graecus* 283 (coll. 631) below (p. 111) (*Census*: 328, nr [1657]).

De morbis popularibus I et III.

Venedig, Bibl. Nazionale Marciana, graecus, 269; s. XI.
Now *graecus* 269 (coll. 533) (*Census*: 329, nr [1662]).
See also (possibly) **[Marcian.]** (p. 108) and **[Marcian. (?)]** above.

(f. 1v) *Laterculi antiqui* (Wie im Vatic. 277 [above p. 101]. Ed. Ilb. – Kühlew. ibid. p. XIX sq.).
(f. 12) *Iusiurandum.*
(f. 12) *Lex.*
(f. 12v) *De arte.*
(f. 16) *De prisca medicina.*
(f. 23v) *Praeceptiones.*
(f. 26) *De decenti ornatu.*
(f. 28) *De natura hominis.*
(f. 33v) *De salubri diaeta.*
(f. 35v) *De genitura.*
(f. 38v) *De natura pueri.*
(f. 47) *De articulis.*
(f. 74) *De humoribus.*
(f. 77v) *De alimento.*
(f. 79v) *De ulceribus.*
(f. 84v) *De morbo sacro.*
(f. 91) *De morbis I.*
(f. 102) *De morbis II et III.*
(f. 129) *De morbis liber IV.*
(f. 154) *De internis affectionibus.*
(f. 142v) *De affectionibus.*
(f. 179) *De victus ratione I–III.*
(f. 208) *De insomniis.*

(f. 211^{v}) *De visu.*
(f. 212^{v}) *De diebus iudicatoriis.*
(f. 215) *Aphorismi.*
(f. 228) *Prognosticon.*
(f. 237^{v}) *De diaeta (regimine) acutorum.*
(f. 257) *De flatibus.*
(f. 261^{v}) *Vectiarius.*
(f. 270) *De ossium natura.*
(f. 275^{v}) *De fracturis.*
(f. 293 B^{v}) *De officina medici.*
(f. 297) *De exsectione foetus. De exsectione pueri* (I).
(f. 298) *De mulierum affectibus.*
(f. 368^{v}) *De sterilibus.*
(f. 379^{v}) *De superfoetatione.*
(f. 385) *De septimestri partu.*
(f. 388) *De octimestri partu.*
(f. 389) *De virginum morbis.*
(f. 390) *De natura muliebri.*
(f. 409) *De morbis popularibus II. IV–VII* (Libri II. IV. V init. desunt).
(f. 446) *Epistulae.*

Galenos, *Linguarum sive dictionum exoletarum Hippocratis explicatio.*
Soranus, *Hippocratis genus et vita secundum Soranum.*

Venedig, Bibl. Nazionale Marciana, graecus, 277; a. 1416, s. XV.
Now *graecus* 277 (coll. 630) (*Census*: 330, nr [1672]).

Galenos:
In Hippocratis vel Polybi opus de salubri victus ratione privatorum commentarius (sine titulo).
Hippocratis aphorismi et Galeni in eos commentarii VII.

Venedig, Bibl. Nazionale Marciana, graecus, 278; s. XI.
Now *graecus* 278 (coll. 873) (*Census*: 330, nr [1673]).

Galenos:
(f. 1) *Hippocratis aphorismi et Galeni in eos commentarii VII.*
(f. 146) *In Hippocratis vel Polybi opus de salubri victus ratione privatorum commentarius.*

Venedig, Bibl. Nazionale Marciana, graecus, 279; s. XV.
Now *graecus* 279 (coll. 705) (*Census*: 330, nr [1674]).

Galenos:
(f. 84^{v}–130^{v}) *In Hippocratis de articulis librum commentarii IV.*
(f. 130^{v}–163^{v}) *In Hippocratis librum de fracturis commentarii III.*
(f. 163^{v}–202) *In Hippocratis librum de officina medici commentarii III.*

Venedig, Bibl. Nazionale Marciana, graecus, 281; s. XV.
Now *graecus* 281 (coll. 581) (*Census*: 331, nr [1677]).

Galenos:
(f. 2–46^{v}) *In Hippocratis librum de acutorum victu commentarii IV.*
(f. 47–71^{v}) *In Hippocratis praedictionum librum primum commentarii III.*

Venedig, Bibl. Nazionale Marciana, graecus, 282; s. XV.
Now *graecus* 282 (coll. 648) (*Census*: 331, nr [1678]).

De genitura.

Galenos:
Galeni in Hippocratis de natura hominis lib. commentarii II.
In Hippocratis vel Polybi opus de salubri victus ratione privatorum commentarius.
(f. 53^{v}–85^{v}) *In Hippocratis prognosticum commentarii III.*

Venedig, Bibl. Nazionale Marciana, graecus, 283; s. XV.
Now *graecus* 283 (coll. 631) (*Census*: 331, nr [1680]).
See also (possibly) **[Marcian., ap. Montfaucon, I, 472]** above (p. 109).

Galenos: (f. 1) *In Hippocratis epidemiarum libros commentarii* (in libr. VI).

Venedig, Bibl. Nazionale Marciana, graecus, 285; s. XV.
Now *graecus* 285 (coll. 708) (*Census*: 332, nr [1683]).

Galenos:
In Hippocratis vel Polybi opus de salubri victus ratione privatorum commentarius.
Hippocratis aphorismi et Galeni in eos commentarii VII.
In Hippocratis epidemiarum libros commentarii (in libr. III).

Venedig, Bibl. Nazionale Marciana, graecus, 296; s. XV.
Now *graecus* 296 (coll. 632) (*Census*: 333, nr [1694]).

De genitura.

Venedig, Bibl. Nazionale Marciana, graecus, 609; XVI.
Now *graecus* 609 (coll. 686) (*Census*: 334, nr [1707]).

Epistulae.

Venedig, Bibl. Nazionale Marciana, appendix graeca
Now Venezia, Biblioteca Nazionale Marciana, *appendix graeca*

Venedig, Bibl. Nazionale Marciana, appendix graeca, V, 4; s. XV.
Now *app. gr.* V.4 (coll. 544) (*Census*: 335, nr [1713]).

Galenos, *In Hippocratis librum de acutorum victu commentarii IV.*

Venedig, Bibl. Nazionale Marciana, appendix graeca, V, 5; s. XV.
Now *app. gr.* V.5 (coll. 1053) (*Census*: 335, nr [1714]).

Galenos:
(f. 2) *Hippocratis aphorismi et Galeni in eos commentarii VII.*
(f. 89) *In Hippocratis librum de acutorum victu commentarii IV.*
(f. 145^{v}) *In Hippocratis prognosticum commentarii III.*
(f. 182^{v}) *In Hippocratis praedictionum librum primum commentarii III* (Commentarius duplex).
(f. 249) *In Hippocratis epidemiarum libros commentarii* (in libr. II.).
(f. 311) *In Hippocratis epidemiarum libros commentarii* (in libr. III. libri II.).

Venedig, Bibl. Nazionale Marciana, appendix graeca, V, 9; s. XV.
Now *app. gr.* V.9 (coll. 1017) (*Census*: 335, nr [1718]).

(f. 473) *De natura pueri.*

Galenos:
(f. 1) *Hippocratis aphorismi et Galeni in eos commentarii VII* (Expl. ἴδρως πολύς = K. XVIII A 176).
(f. 508) *In Hippocratis librum de acutorum victu commentarii IV.*

Venedig, Bibl. Nazionale Marciana, appendix graeca, V, 10; s. XVI.
Now app. gr. V.10 (coll. 1444) (*Census*: 335, nr [1719]).

Galenos: (f. 29) *Hippocratis aphorismi et Galeni in eos commentarii VII.*

Venedig, Bibl. Nazionale Marciana, appendix graeca, V, 13; s. XIV–XVI.
Now *app. gr.* V.13 (coll. 1221) (*Census*: 336, nr [1723]).

(f. 118) *De venae sectione.*

Venedig, Bibl. Nazionale Marciana, appendix graeca, V, 14; s. XV.
Now *app. gr.* V.14 (coll. 1408) (*Census*: 336, nr [1725]).
See also **V, 14 (ol. Nanian. 248)** below.

(f. 10) *De visu* (Expl. ἠλαιωμένον ἐγκατακαίειν = L. IX 154, 11).

Venedig, Bibl. Nazionale Marciana, appendix graeca, V, 14 (ol. Nanian. 248); s. XV, XVI.
Same as **V, 14** above.
Now *app. gr.* V.14 (coll. 1408) (*Census*: 336, nr [1726]).

(f. 1) *De insomniis.*
(f. 7) *De diebus iudicatoriis.*
(f. 11) *De aëre, aquis et locis.*
(f. 19) *De genitura.*
(f. 22v) *De superfoetatione* (Expl. βάπτειν δὲ τὰς μήλας = L. VIII 496,9).

Venedig, Bibl. Nazionale Marciana, appendix graeca, V, 15; s. XVI.
Now *app. gr.* V.15 (coll. 1299) (*Census*: 335, nr [1727]).

Galenos, *In Hippocratis epidemiarum libros commentarii* (in libr. I. liber I; Expl. τῶν ἔνδον τοῦ περιτοναίου μορίων; *Das* Expl. *ist vielmehr das von* Comm. III in Epid. Γ'; *vgl. oben* Monac. 231) (see p. 47).
Erotianus, *Vocum Hippocraticarum conlectio.*

Venedig, Bibl. Nazionale Marciana, appendix graeca, V, 16; s. XVI.
Now *app. gr.* V.16 (coll. 1318) (*Census*: 335, nr [1728]).

(f. 82) *Ad Ptolemaeum regem epistula de hominis fabrica.*
(f. 146) *Hippocratis vel Dioclis epistula ad Ptolemaeum Aegyptii regem.*

Venedig, Bibl. Nazionale Marciana, appendix graeca, V, 19; s. –, XV.
Now *app. gr.* V.19 (coll. 986) (*Census*: 335, nr [1730]).

(f. 475) *De natura hominis.*

Venedig, Bibl. S. Anton.

[Venedig, Bibl. S. Anton.].
Now Wien, Österreichische Nationalbibliothek, *historicus graecus* 130 below (p. 115) (*Census*: 337, nr [1735]).

Aphorismi.

[Venedig, Bibl. S. Anton.].
Now Paris, Bibliothèque nationale de France, *graecus* 2253 above (p. 76) (*Census*: 337, nr [1736]).

De humoribus.

Wien, Bibl. Colleg. S. J. Rossianus

Wien, Bibl. Colleg. S. J. Rossianus, XI.167; s. XV.
Now *Vaticanus Rossianus* 982 (*Census*: 348, nr [1742]).

(f. 7^{v}) *De quattuor elementis et humoribus naturae hominis* (Ἱπποκράτους περὶ τῶν δ' στοιχείων καὶ χυμῶν δι' ὧν συνίσταται ὁ ἄνθρωπος. Inc. Ἰστέον ὅτι ὁ ἄνθρωπος συνίσταται. Expl. f. 9^{v} ὅσα δὲ γένηται ἐν χειμῶνι ἀπαλλάσσονται).
(f. 9^{v}) *Ad Ptolemaeum regem epistula de hominis fabrica* (Ἐκ τῶν τοῦ ἱπποκράτους περὶ τεσσάρων στοιχείων. Inc. συνέστηκεν ὁ κόσμος ἐκ. Expl. 11^{v} εἰσέρχεται εἰς τὴν κύστιν τὸ ὕδωρ = p. 279–285 Ermerins. Folgt f. 11^{v} περὶ αἰσθήσεων. Inc. αἰσθητήρια δὲ ἐστὶν. Expl. f. 12^{r} ὄνυχες δὲ ψυχρᾶς καὶ ξηρᾶς κράσεως εἰσὶν = p. 287, 1–289, 6 Ermerins).
(f. 12^{v}) *De septimanis* (Inc. ἰστέον ὡς ἱπποκράτης ἑπτὰ ἡλικίας. Expl. ibid. γέρων εἰς τὰς δεκατέσσαρας ἑβδομάδας).

Wien, Gollob Privatbesitz

Wien, Gollob Privatbesitz, Vindob.; s. XV.
Now Wien, Österreichische Nationalbibliothek, *Supplementum graecum* 179 (*Census*: 348–349, nr [1743]).

Epistulae (Epp. 1–9. 25. 10–16. 18. 20. 19. 21. 17. 22–24).

Wien, Hofbibliothek, Vindob./Vindobon.
Now Wien, Österreichische Nationalbibliothek, *Vindobonenses*

[Wien, Hofbibliothek, Vindob. Lamb. VI 85].
Same as **Wien, Hofbibliothek, Vindob. med. 4** below (p. 116) (*Census*: 351, nr [1746])
= Wien, Österreichische Nationalbibliothek, *medicus graecus* 4.

De diaeta (regimine) acutorum.

[Wien, Hofbibliothek, Vindob. ap. Nessel P. III].
= Wien, Österreichische Nationalbibliothek, *medicus graecus* 15.

Galenos, *In Hippocratis librum de acutorum victu commentarii IV.*

Wien, Hofbibliothek, Vindobon. 69 B 101.
= *69.B.101 (*Census*: 355, nr [1758]).

»Handschriftliche Bemerkungen aus einer Basileens. des Hipp., dem Handexemplar des Cornarius. Zu περὶ διαίτης p. 81–109 Bas., zu π. ἱερῆς νούσου p. 122–128«.

[Wien, Hofbibliothek, Vindob., 179].
Possibly same as Wien, Hofbibliothek, Vindob. med. 15 (*Census*: 356, nr [1761]).
= ? Wien, Österreichische Nationalbibliothek, *medicus graecus* 15.

Prognostica (*Wie im* Taurin. [C VI 21 9b VI 18]) (p. 108).

Wien, Hofbibliothek, histor. 130; s. XV–XVI.
See also **[Venedig, Bibl. S. Anton.]** above (p. 114).

(f. 182–200) *Aphorismi* (Expl. ὅταν ὁμοῦ τε πῦον καὶ χολὴν ἀναβήσσῃ).

Wien, Hofbibliothek, Vindob. lat. 4772 (tab. cod. III 382); s. XV.
Latin manuscript (*Census*: 357, nr [1765]).

(f. 9) *Aphorismi* (Expl. ξβ'. ἐπὶ σφακελισμοῦ ἀπόστασις ὀστέου).
(f. 105) *Iusiurandum.*

Wien, Hofbibliothek, Vindob. med. 4; s. X.
See also **[Vindob. Lamb. VI 85]** above (p. 115).

(f. 1) *De internis affectionibus* (Inc. L. VII 168, 4 ⟨περιστρέ⟩φηται).
(f. 46) *De affectionibus.*
(f. 72) *De morbo sacro.*
(f. 88) *De morbis I.*
(f. 88) *De morbis II et III.*
(f. 174ᵛ) *De victus ratione I–III.*
(f. 233) *De insomniis.*
(f. 241) *De mulierum affectibus* (Expl. pro διακλυζέσθω sic: διανιζέσθω ὃς ἂν περὶ ἰήσιος ἐθέλῃ ἐρωτᾶν: – γυναικείων β'. *Vgl.* Περὶ νούσων lib. I in.).
(f. 383ᵛ) *De natura muliebri* (Expl. προνη⟨στεύσασαν⟩ = L. VII 412, 16).

Wien, Hofbibliothek, Vindob. med. 8; s. XV.
See also **[8]** (possibly) below.

(f. 282) *Sententiae de vita et morte* (Inc. wie im Lond. Medical Society [AA a 1 = Xa 32] [above p. 35]. Expl. εἰς ἓξ ἡμέρας ἀποθανεῖται).

[Wien, Hofbibliothek, Vindob. med. 8].
Possibly same as **Wien, Hofbibliothek, Vindob. med. 8** above (*Census*: 358, nr [1772]).
= ? *medicus graecus* 8.

Excerpta varia.

Wien, Hofbibliothek, Vindob. med. 13; s. –, XV.

(f. 1) *De genitura* (Inscr. Περὶ γεννήσεως ἀνθρώπου καὶ περὶ γονῆς. Inc. Νόμος μέν. Expl. f. 4ᵛ ταῦτα αἰσχυνόμεθα καὶ κρύπτειν σπουδάζομεν).
(f. 4ᵛ–6ᵛ) *Hippocratis et Galeni philosophia de natura hominis.*
(f. 59–128) *Jatrosophium* (Ἰατροσόφ. Ἱππ.).

Wien, Hofbibliothek, Vindob. med. 14; s. –, XVI.

Jatrosophium.
(f. 47) *De exsectione foetus. De exsectione pueri* (II).

[Wien, Hofbibliothek, Vindob. med. 15].
Possibly same as Wien, Hofbibliothek, Vindob. med. 15 (*Census*: 358, nr [1779]).
= ? *medicus graecus* 15.

Excerpta varia.

Wien, Hofbibliothek, Vindob. med. 16; s. XV–XVI.
s. XV.
See also **med. 16 (ol. 35)** below.

(f. 1) *De venae sectione.*

Theophilus, *Commentarius in Hippocratis aphorismos* (Expl. δηλοῖ γὰρ ἐπίτασιν ξηρότητος. *Abschrift im Berol. fol. 39 [275]* [above p. 10]).
Stephanus Atheniensis: (f. 185) *In aphorismos Hippocratis commentarius* (Sine auctoris nomine. Σχόλια εἰς τοὺς Ἱππ. ἀφορ. κατὰ σύνοψιν. Inc. Ὅρος ἀφορισμοῦ. Ἀφορισμός ἐστι λόγος σύντομος. Expl. δηλοῖ γὰρ ἐπίτασιν ξηρότητος).

Wien, Hofbibliothek, Vindob. med. 16 (ol. 35); s. –, XV.
Same as **16** above (*Census*: 358–359, nr [1781]).
= *medicus graecus* 16.

(f. 185–201 [marg.]) *Prognosticon.*

Wien, Hofbibliothek, Vindob. med. 24; s. XV.

(f. 1) *De morbo sacro.*
(f. 2) *Epistulae* (Ep. 1 etc.; expl. f. 3^{v} ὧν ὁ δι' ἀρετῆς ὑποκαθαρθεὶς ὑγιάζεται ἐγὼ δὴ ...).

Wien, Hofbibliothek, Vindob. med. 28; s. –, XV.
See also **med. [28 (?)]** below.

(f. 140–156^{v}) *Aphorismi* (Expl. ξε'. ἐπὶ λευκῷ φλέγματι ὕδρωψ ἐπιγίνεται).

[Wien, Hofbibliothek, Vindob. med. 28 (?); s. XV].
Same as **28** above (*Census*: 360, nr [1793]).
= *medicus graecus* 28.

De humoribus (Frgm. Π. χ. ἐκ τῶν Ἱππ.).

Wien, Hofbibliothek, Vindob. med. 31; s. –, XV ex.
s. XV.

(f. 166^{v}) *Aphorismi* (I 1.2 = L. IV 458, 1–12).

Wien, Hofbibliothek, Vindob. med. 32; s. XVI.

(f. 11) *Testamentum.*

Wien, Hofbibliothek, Vindob. med. 34; s. –.
= *Par. suppl. gr. 447.*
Now Paris, Bibliothèque nationale de France, *Supplementum graecum* 447 above (p. 89) (*Census*: 360, nr [1798]).

Galenos :
In Hippocratis de natura hominis lib. commentarii II.
(f. 1) *Hippocratis aphorismi et Galeni in eos commentarii VII.*
(f. 229) *In Hippocratis vel Polybi opus de salubri victus ratione privatorum commentarius.*

Wien, Hofbibliothek, Vindob. med. 38 ^{c}; s. –.

Erotianus, *Vocum Hippocraticarum conlectio.*

Wien, Hofbibliothek, Vindob. med. 40; s. XV.

(f. 125) *Ad Ptolemaeum regem epistula de hominis fabrica* (Expl. ὁ μὲν ἔξωθεν νευρώδης, ὁ δὲ ἔνδοθεν σαρκώδης).

Wien, Hofbibliothek, Vindob. med. 41; s. XIV.
s. XIV–XV.
See also (possibly) **[41]** below.

(f. 81 [f. 81^{r}–82^{r}]) *De quattuor elementis et humoribus naturae hominis* (Inc. Ἰστέον ὅτι ὁ ἄνθρωπος συνίσταται ἐκ τεσσάρων στοιχείων. Expl. εἰς τὰς τέσσαρας ἑβδομάδας. *Wie im* Vindob. Rossian [XI. 167] [above p. 114]).
(f. 82^{r}–83^{r}; 83^{r}–83^{v}) *Ad Ptolemaeum regem epistula de hominis fabrica* (*Wie im* Vindob. Rossian. [XI. 167]).
(f. 83^{v}) *De septimanis* (*Wie im* Vindob. Rossian. [XI. 167]).

[Wien, Hofbibliothek, Vindob. med. 41].
Possibly same **as 41** above.
= ? *medicus graecus* 41 (*Census*: 361, nr [1805]).

Excerpta varia.

Wien, Hofbibliothek, Vindob. med. 43; s. XVI.

Erotianus: (f. 83–121v) *Vocum Hippocraticarum conlectio.*
Soranus: (f. 122) *Hippocratis genus et vita secundum Soranum* (Inc. Πρῶτον τὴν ἐπωνυμίαν. Expl. ἐν περιόδοισιν ὅτι ἑβδομήκοντα κινέεται. »Wahrscheinlich nicht hierhergehörig.« Schoene).

Wien, Hofbibliothek, Vindob. med. 44; s. XV.XVI, XV–XVI.

(f. 232–304v) *Prognosticon* (Sine auct. nomine. Expl. τεσσαρακοστὴν ἑξηκοστὴν ὅρον ἱστάμενος).

Stephanus Atheniensis: (f. 1) *In aphorismos Hippocratis commentarius* (Inc. ἐν τῇσι = Dietz p. 283, 3).
Theophilus: (f. 1–126v) *Commentarius in Hippocratis aphorismos* (*Vgl.* Stephanus).
Galenos: (f. 232) *In Hippocratis prognosticum commentarii III.*

Wien, Hofbibliothek, Vindob. med. 47; s. XV, XVI.

(f. 432) *De ulceribus.*

Wien, Hofbibliothek, Vindob. med. 48; s. XIV–XV.

(f. 172–196) *Aphorismi* (Expl. τὰ καταμήνια ταύτῃ ἐκλέλοιπεν. γυναιξὶν ὁκόσῃισιν ἐντὸς μα... L. IV 544, 15. 16 ?).

Wien, Hofbibliothek, Vindob. med. 49; s. XVI.

(f. 2–21) *Aphorismi* (Expl. εὐνοῦχοι οὔτε ποδαγριῶσιν οὔτε φαλακροὶ γίγνονται L. IV 570, 5).

Wien, Hofbibliothek, Vindob. med. 52; s. –, XV.

(f. 49–55) *Epistula ad Ptolemaeum regem de sanitate tuenda* (᾽Εγκύκλιος ἐπιστ. Ἱππ. πρὸς Πτολ. βασ., ὅπως ἐπεισέρχεται τῷ τοῦ ἀνθρώπου σώματι νόσος. Expl. μάλιστα θαρρούντων τῷ ἔθει).

(f. 67) *Ad Ptolemaeum regem epistula de hominis fabrica* (Inc. ψυχρά · τὸ δὲ ὕδωρ ψυχρὸν καὶ ὑγρόν. Expl. ἐπὶ τὰς ἁπλᾶς καὶ ἡνωμένας τοῦ νοῦ θεωρίας ἀναγομένη).
(f. 84–92) *Excerpta varia* (Inc. *wie im* [Vatic.] Palat. 400 [above p. 96]. Expl. ἕνωσον καὶ χρῆσαι).

Wien, Hofbibliothek, Vindob. med. 53; s. XVI.
See also (possibly) **[53]** below.

(f. 8ᵛ–10ᵛ) *Testamentum.*
(f. 59ᵛ–128ᵛ) *Jatrosophium* (Inc. f. 70 περὶ ἀπηγάνου εἰς κρίον α̅. Expl. δὸς πιεῖν μετὰ οἴνου καὶ ὠφελεῖται: – τέλος τῶν οκβ' κεφαλαίων).

[Wien, Hofbibliothek, Vindob. med. 53].
Possibly same as **53** above (*Census*: 362, nr [1817]).
= ? *medicus graecus* 53.

Excerpta varia.

Wien, Hofbibliothek, Vindob. phil. 74; s. XVI.
Now philos. et philol. gr. 74 (*Census*: 362: nr [1820]).

Theophilus: (f. 52–107v) *Commentarius in Hippocratis aphorismos* (Expl. πάντως ἂν εἴη ἴαμα. Vgl. Oxford [Bodl.] Roe 14 [above p. 53]).

Wien, Hofbibliothek, Vindob. phil. 82; s. XV–XVI.
Now *philos. et philol. gr.* 82 (*Census*: 362: nr [1821]).

(f. 158ᵛ–177) *Epistulae* (Epp. 1–22 ?).

Wien, Hofbibliothek, Vindob. phil. 178; s. XV.
Now *philos. et philol. gr.* 178 (*Census*: 362: nr [1823]).

(f. 43ʳ–43ᵛ) *De sudoribus* (Inc. Οἱ δ' ἱδρῶτες ἄριστοι μέν εἰσιν ἐν ἅπασι τοῖσιν ὀξέοισιν. Expl. πίστει καὶ πόθῳ δοξάζωμεν).
(f. 345) *Epistula ad Ptolemaeum regem de sanitate tuenda* (Expl. εὖ διάξεις, μέγιστε βασιλεῦ Πτολεμαῖε).

Wien, Hofbibliothek, Vindob. phil. 179; s. XV.
Same as **philos. et philol. 179** below.
Now *philos. et philol. gr.* 179 (*Census*: 362: nr [1824]).

(f. 123ᵛ) *Aphorismi* (π. καιρ. πρόγνωσις = Aph. III 11–14 L. IV 490–492).

Wien, Hofbibliothek, Vindob. phil. 192; s. XV.
Now *philos. et philol. gr.* 192 (*Census*: 362: nr [1826]).

(f. 112) *De insomniis* (Inc. Ὁκόσα τῶν ἐνυπνίων).

Wien, Hofbibliothek, Vindob. phil. 219; s. XV.
Now *philos. et philol. gr.* 219 (*Census*: 362: nr [1827]).

(f. 140) *Iusiurandum.*

Wien, Hofbibliothek, Vindob. philos. et philol. 179; s. XV.
See also **phil. 179** above.

(f. 123^{v}) *De IV aetatibus praenotio.*

Wien, Hofbibliothek, Vindob. theol. 293; s. XVI.

(f. 92) *Ad Ptolemaeum regem epistula de hominis fabrica.*

Wolfenbüttel, Bibl. Guelf. August.
Now Wolfenbüttel, Herzog August Bibliothek Wolfenbüttel

[Wolfenbüttel, Bibl. Guelf. August., August. 18, 1, –].
Now 18.1 Aug. 4to (*Census*: 369, nr [1839]).
See also **3132 (18.1 Aug. 4°)** below.

Epistulae (? Ep. ad Hystan.).

Wolfenbüttel, Bibl. Guelf., Guelferb. 3132 (18.1 Aug. 4°); s. XV.
Same as **[August. 18, 1]** above.
= 18.1 Aug. 4to (*Census*: 369, nr [1840]).

(f. 115–116) *Epistulae* (Epp. 1–3. 5).

Zaragoza

Zaragoza, Bibl. d. Cat. d. Pil., 1115 (olim 1427); s. XVI.
Now New Haven, Yale University, Harvey Cushing/John Hay Whitney Medical Library, Manuscript 50 vault (*Census*: 372–373, nr [1856]).

Damascius: (f. 1) *Expositio in Prognostica Hippocratis. Sectiones II.*

Zürich, Stadtbibliothek
Now Zürich, Zentralbibliothek Zürich – Kantons-, Stadt- und Universitätsbibliothek

Zürich, Stadtbibliothek, C 136; s. XVI.
Now MS. C 136 (*Census*: 373, nr [1859]).

(f. 117) *De partibus hominis* (de partibus hominis).
(f. 177) *De generatione hominis*.

www.ingramcontent.com/pod-product-compliance
Ingram Content Group UK Ltd.
Pitfield, Milton Keynes, MK11 3LW, UK
UKHW050953290926
15470UKWH00006B/1798

9 783110 600674